I0765368

Free Gift

Sign up to my mailing list to receive this FREE
exclusive copy of

5 Step. 5 Minute Balance Exercises For Seniors Over 80 - The 1st 7 Days

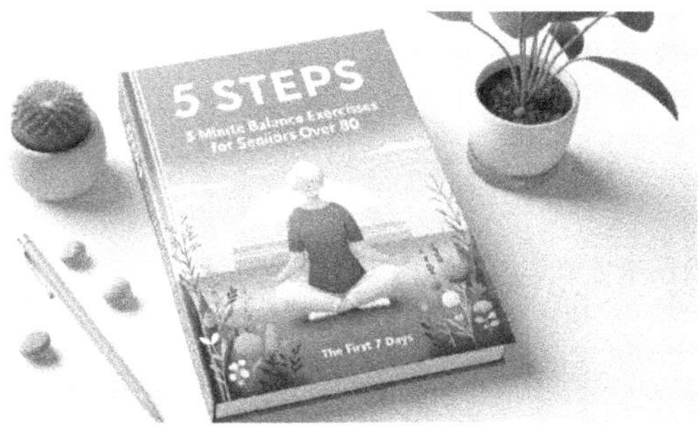

As well as to be notified on any new releases,
giveaways, contests, cover reveals and so much more.

Click here to sign up for my newsletter

Description

"Stop Glue Ear: A Step by Step Guide For All Ages"

Your Compass to Navigating and Conquering Glue Ear

Are you or a loved one grappling with the discomfort of glue ear? This authoritative guide by Jagoda E. Handor demystifies this common yet misunderstood condition, offering a beacon of hope and clarity for those affected.

Inside, You'll Discover:

- Deep Insights: Understand the symptoms and causes of glue ear, a condition that crosses age boundaries, from infants to seniors.
- Holistic Approaches: Explore a range of treatments — from tried-and-tested medical interventions to innovative, natural remedies.
- Empowering Strategies: Learn practical, daily tips and techniques to manage and prevent glue ear, enhancing your quality of life.
- Expert Guidance: Benefit from the author's rich blend of personal experiences and professional insights, offering a unique and relatable perspective.

This book is more than a guide; it's a journey towards better ear health.

Embrace the opportunity to transform the challenges of glue ear into a dialogue of care. "Stop Glue Ear" is your guide to turning whispers of discomfort into a story of understanding and resilience.

- *"As someone who has struggled with glue ear for years, 'Stop Glue Ear' has been a game-changer. The book's comprehensive approach and practical tips have significantly improved my quality of life. It's a must-read for anyone dealing with this condition." - Emily R., Long-time Glue Ear Sufferer*
- *"Jagoda E. Handor's guide is insightful and empathetic. It was enlightening to read about glue ear from both a personal and professional perspective. This book is a valuable resource for healthcare professionals and patients alike." - Dr. Aiden Smith, ENT Specialist*
- *"This book was a lifeline for our family. Understanding and managing our child's glue ear became so much easier. The blend of medical information and real-life tips is perfect for any parent navigating this journey." - Sarah and Michael Johnson, Parents of a Child with Glue Ear*

Chapter 1: Introduction to Glue Ear

Enter the intriguing world of glue ear, a condition that affects all ages. Up when you have a cold? Or noticed a child tugging at their ear with a pained expression? They might surpass mere fleeting discomforts. Overlooking the glue ear can cause these discomforts.

In the sanctuary of our daily lives, glue ear lurks unnoticed, affecting people from the playful toddler to the wise senior. Its name might conjure up images of craft projects gone awry, but the reality is far more profound. Glue ear occurs when a sticky fluid, much like glue, accumulates in the middle ear. This fluid can muffle sounds, like listening through a foggy mist, and for some, it leads to a haunting silence as it dampens the vibrant symphony of life.

But what causes this fluid to gather where it doesn't belong? Often, it's an aftermath of infections, allergies, or even changes in air pressure. For others, it's a puzzle, with pieces hidden in genetics or environmental factors. Ear problems aren't limited to childhood; glue ear can affect anyone. It can be a silent visitor in adults and seniors, bringing a unique set of challenges and concerns.

In this chapter, we embark on a journey to demystify the glue ear. We'll untangle the web of symptoms that range from a slight hearing loss to feel fullness in the ears, akin to being underwater. We'll explore the twists and turns of how a glue ear can affect different people in different ways–from a minor annoyance to a significant barrier in communication and quality of life.

Our goal is to empower, not just inform, by unraveling the layers of the glue ear. Understanding the glue ear is the first step towards managing it, especially in the fog of uncertainty. Whether you're a concerned parent, an individual experiencing symptoms, or just curious about this common condition, this chapter is your gateway to a clearer understanding.

So, let us begin this journey with open minds and attentive ears. Let's explore the mysterious world of glue ear together, uncovering its secrets and learning how to navigate its challenges. Welcome to the first step in a journey towards clarity, both in hearing and

Symptoms and Diagnosis

Ever constantly ask people to repeat themselves, or feeling like your ears are underwater? What might seem like minor nuisances could whisper a deeper story–the story of a glue ear.

This chapter explores symptoms and diagnosis, where understanding signs is vital for effective care. The mundane or fleeting. It begins–feel a fullness in the ears, akin to the pressure you feel when flying or diving deep underwater. Some describe it as having cotton wool in their ears, a muffled, distant sound that turns life's melody into a muted hum.

For the little ones, it might manifest in behaviors rather than words–increased irritability, difficulty in responding to sounds, or frequent ear tugging. In adults, maybe an elusive decline in hearing, often shrugged off as just another sign of aging. However, the glue ear goes beyond hearing issues. It can be a silent disruptor in classrooms and workplaces, a barrier in conversations and connections.

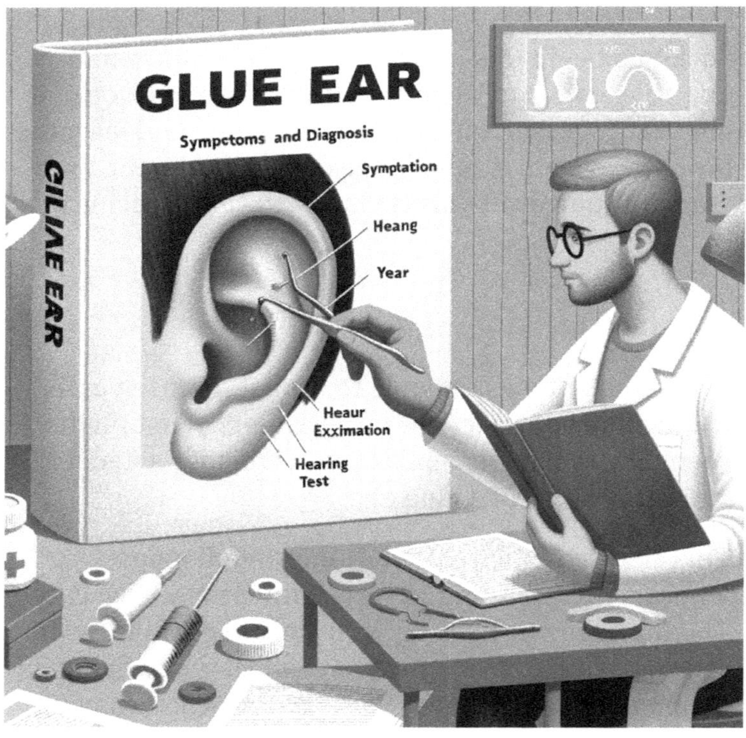

Diagnosing the glue ear is akin to piecing together a puzzle. It's not just about what we hear, but also about what we see. Doctors often use an otoscope, a tool that lights up the hidden world inside our ears, revealing the state of the eardrum and any unusual fluid behind it. Sometimes, an audiogram might join the diagnostic dance, measuring the softest sounds one can hear, mapping out the peaks and valleys of hearing loss.

But what happens when the usual tools don't draw the full picture? Some professionals, especially in challenging or borderline cases, may use a tympano gram. This test checks how well the eardrum can move, offering clues about any stubborn fluid in the middle ear.

As we navigate through the maze of symptoms and diagnostic tools, our journey is lit by a simple yet powerful truth.–knowledge is the key. Understanding the signs and the pathways to diagnosis empowers us to seek timely help, to turn the whispers of discomfort into a dialogue for care.

By the end of this chapter, the once murky waters of glue ear symptoms and diagnosis will clear, offering you a lens to view, understand, and act. It's a step towards demystifying this silent visitor, towards clarity not just in hearing, but in knowledge and action.

Chapter 2: Glue Ear Across Different Age Groups

Infants and Toddlers

In the enchanting yet complex world of infants and toddlers, glue ear often creeps in silently, an unbidden guest in the developing landscape of their tiny ears. In these early, formative years, the Eustachian tubes – the vital passageways that connect the middle ear to the back of the nose – are still maturing. This makes them more susceptible to blockages, setting the stage for glue ear to take hold.

For the keen observer, the symptoms of glue ear in these younglings are a silent language waiting to be deciphered. These little ones, with their unformed words and uncharted expressions, can't verbalize the discomfort brewing inside their ears. Instead, their behavior becomes the canvas of symptoms – increased irritability that seems unexplained, a disturbed sleep pattern that disrupts the peaceful lullabies of the night, or a sudden reluctance to engage in playful babbles.

During feeding times, you might notice an infant's growing fussiness, or a struggle to suckle – both subtle cries for help from the discomfort in their ears. As they grow into the toddler stage, their responses to sounds may dwindle, their once eager reactions to familiar voices and melodies fading into a concerning quietude.

The ramifications of glue ear in this tender phase of life are profound. It's not just about the ears; it's about the cascading effect on language development and social interaction. These early years are critical for speech and language acquisition, and glue ear can cast a shadow on this vital developmental milestone. A child's ability to hear clearly is the cornerstone of learning to speak, to communicate, and to interact with the world.

The role of vigilant parenting becomes paramount in early detection. It's a role that demands patience, observation, and a keen sense of awareness to the unspoken. The 'wait and see' approach often becomes the initial path of action, as many cases of glue ear in infants and toddlers resolve naturally over time. This period of watchful waiting is not about inaction; it's about understanding the natural course of the condition and giving the little one's body a chance to resolve it on its own.

However, if the whispers of glue ear linger, turning into a more persistent guest, medical intervention might come into play. The insertion of ear tubes – tiny cylinders placed through the eardrum to ventilate the middle ear and drain the fluid – becomes a consideration. This procedure, often quick and with minimal discomfort, can be a doorway to relief, releasing the pressure and the fluid that muffled the vibrant world of sounds for the child.

In the journey of tackling glue ear in infants and toddlers, the goal is clear – to ensure that these young explorers of life do not miss the symphony of sounds that surround them. It's about safeguarding their right to hear, to speak, and to engage with the world in its fullest melody.

School-Age Children

In the vibrant, often chaotic world of school, where learning and play intertwine, glue ear can silently erect walls around a child, walls that distort and dampen the sounds of their environment. For school-age children, the journey through classrooms and playgrounds can become a labyrinth of challenges if glue ear steps in unnoticed.

The symptoms in these young learners can be as diverse as their personalities. For some, it's the struggle to hear over the din of a noisy classroom, their faces a mask of concentration as they try to catch the drifting words of teachers and classmates. Others might find themselves visiting the school nurse more often than their peers, battling ear infections that seem to come and go like uninvited guests. And then there are those whose academic performance begins to wane, not because of a lack of effort or intelligence, but because the clarity of sound that carries knowledge has become muffled.

But glue ear is more than just an ailment of the ears; it's a ripple that touches every aspect of a child's school life. It can lurk behind difficulties in social interactions, behind the moments of frustration and confusion when words get lost in the fog of impaired hearing. This condition can be a silent thief, stealing away the joys of learning and the ease of communication.

Recognizing and managing glue ear in school-age children requires a symphony of approaches. Regular hearing assessments become a cornerstone of this strategy, a way to catch the whispers of glue ear before they turn into shouts. For some children, the path to clearer hearing might involve the use of hearing aids or the placement of temporary ear tubes, small interventions that can open up a world of sound.

But the melody of management isn't just medical. It's also about the harmonious adaptations in their daily environments. At home, it might mean creating quieter spaces for study and rest, or ensuring that communication is clear and visual cues are used. In the classroom, it's about the thoughtful accommodations – seating the child closer to the teacher, away from the noisy distractions of open windows or bustling hallways. It's about inclusive teaching methods, where every child's need is acknowledged and catered to, where learning is not just a privilege of the perfectly hearing.

In this chapter, we explore these diverse strategies, painting a picture of a world where glue ear doesn't have to be a barrier. It's a world where understanding, adaptation, and timely medical care harmonize to create an environment where every child can thrive, where the sound of their laughter and learning rings clear and unimpeded.

In the vibrant tapestry of adolescence and young adulthood, a time bursting with dreams, social exploration, and self-discovery, glue ear can be an unexpected and formidable adversary. Although less common in this age group, when it does make an appearance, its impact can be deeply profound, sending ripples through the delicate process of forging identities and connections.

The manifestation of glue ear in teens and young adults can be a subtle invader. It may begin as a gradual hearing loss, the soft notes of life's soundtrack fading into a distant hum. Or it might be the persistent sensation of fullness in the ear, a constant reminder that something isn't quite right. These seemingly minor symptoms can be the stealthy culprits behind larger challenges – a hesitancy to engage in conversations, a withdrawal from social gatherings, or an uncharacteristic dip in academic performance.

This phase of life is a critical one, where each experience is a building block in the towering structure of self-identity. Glue ear, with its ability to muffle not just sound but also the confidence and ease of social interactions, can become a significant obstacle. The path to navigating friendships and educational pursuits becomes clouded, as the clarity of communication is dimmed.

Addressing glue ear in this demographic is not just about medical treatment; it's about empowering these young individuals. It's about arming them with the knowledge and tools to proactively manage their condition, to reclaim the clarity of sound and confidence. Treatment may often step into more advanced territories, like sophisticated hearing aids designed to blend seamlessly with their lifestyle, or medical interventions that address the root cause of the condition.

Beyond the realm of medical solutions, there's an equally important aspect of support – maintaining social engagement and mental well-being. It involves encouraging open conversations about their challenges, fostering an environment where they feel heard and supported, not just in the physical sense but emotionally too. It's about providing platforms and opportunities for them to engage, to connect, and to thrive, not in spite of their condition, but alongside it.

In this chapter, we explore the multifaceted approach to managing glue ear in teens and young adults. It's a journey of empowerment, a narrative that intertwines medical solutions with strategies for mental and social well-being. It's about ensuring that this pivotal chapter in their lives is not defined by what they struggle to hear, but by how they choose to respond and grow.

Adults and Seniors

In the tapestry of adult and senior life, where every experience is a thread woven into the fabric of memory and wisdom, glue ear can be a silent, unnoticed thread that subtly alters the pattern. Often dismissed as just another sign of aging, glue ear in adults, and particularly in seniors, can be a significant, yet overlooked, health concern.

The manifestations of glue ear in this age group are as varied as the individuals themselves. For some, it begins as a mild hearing loss, a gradual dimming of the world's auditory vibrancy. Others may experience a constant sensation of ear blockage, an invisible barrier that muffles conversations and distills the richness of sounds into a faint echo. These symptoms, seemingly innocuous at first, can have profound implications. They can amplify the feelings of isolation and loneliness that often accompany older age, turning the golden years into a silent reverie.

Addressing glue ear in adults and seniors is a delicate dance of medical intervention and lifestyle adaptation. Regular hearing check-ups become not just a recommendation but a necessity, a vital tool in detecting and managing glue ear before it deepens its roots. These evaluations offer a window into the health of the ear, helping to distinguish glue ear from other age-related hearing issues.

The management of glue ear at this stage of life often calls for a multifaceted approach. Medications to reduce inflammation may be prescribed, aiming to clear the blockages in the Eustachian tubes. In some cases, minor surgical procedures, like the insertion of ear tubes, offer a more direct solution, providing immediate relief and restoring the clarity of sound.

Hearing aids, too, play a pivotal role. Modern technology has transformed these devices into discreet, powerful tools that not only amplify sound but also enhance the quality of life. They are not just devices; they are gateways to clearer communication, to staying connected with loved ones, and to engaging fully in the world around them.

But beyond medical treatments, lifestyle adaptations are equally important. Creating environments conducive to better hearing, like reducing background noise and using visual cues in communication, can significantly improve daily interactions. It's also about nurturing the emotional well-being, encouraging participation in social activities, and fostering connections that keep the spirit of conversation alive.

In this chapter, we delve into the nuances of managing glue ear in adults and seniors. It's a journey of understanding, of balancing medical solutions with practical, everyday changes. It's about ensuring that the later years of life are not defined by the limitations of glue ear but enriched by the ways it is overcome.

A bonus detailed chapter on over 80's is included at chapter 6. It takes the time to go into more detai. It is perfect, not just for over 80's but anyone of any age who has chronic issues.

Chapter 3: Treatment and Management

Medical Treatments

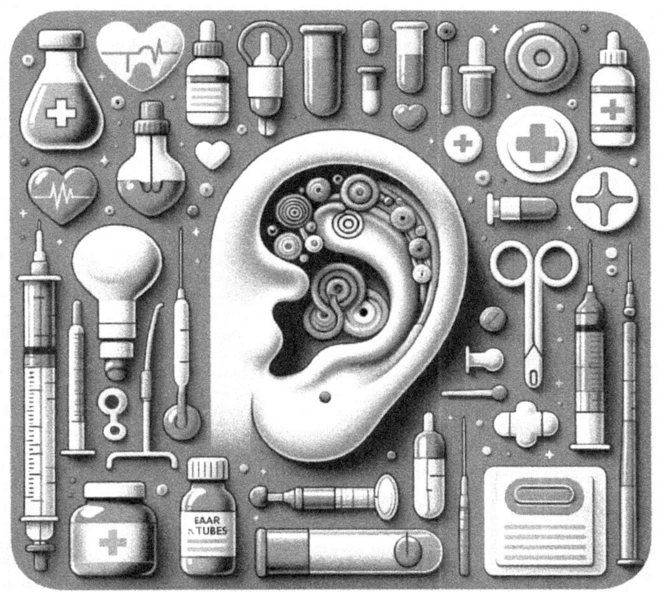

MEDICAL TREATMENTS FOR GLIUE EAR

Navigating the waters of the glue ear, a condition as elusive as it is common, calls for a robust arsenal of medical treatments. Each case of the glue ear is as unique as the individual it affects, requiring a tailored approach to management. This chapter embarks on a deep dive into the array of medical interventions available, demystifying them and presenting them in an approachable and comprehensible manner.

In the battle against the glue ear, antibiotics often take the lead, especially when there is a suspicion of an infection as the underlying cause. These powerful medications work to eliminate the infection, thus reducing the inflammation and the accompanying fluid build-up in the middle ear. However, the use of antibiotics is a delicate balancing act. It requires a judicious assessment of the potential benefits versus the risks, such as antibiotic resistance, ensuring that their prescription is as prudent as it is effective.

When fluid accumulation steadfastly persists, despite initial treatments, ear tubes–also known as grommets–come into play. Surgeons surgically insert these minuscule yet mighty tubes into the eardrum, allowing the trapped fluid to escape from the middle ear. The insertion of ear tubes is a quick procedure, often bringing immediate relief and a significant improvement in hearing, with minimal discomfort involved.

For adults and especially seniors, where the glue ear may present more complex challenges, a more advanced approach may warrant. Myringotomy, a procedure involving a precise incision in the eardrum, allows for the direct drainage of the fluid. Often, doctors combine this procedure with placing ear tubes, providing a more comprehensive solution for individuals dealing with persistent and bothersome symptoms.

In the arena of hearing loss, a frequent companion of the glue ear, hearing aids emerge as invaluable allies.

Modern hearing aids transcend the traditional role of mere sound amplifiers. They are sophisticated devices capable of being finely tuned to meet the specific hearing requirements of the wearer. These devices serve as vital bridges, spanning the gaps in hearing created by glue ear, and restoring a sense of normalcy and connection to the auditory world.

As we traverse the landscape of current treatments, this chapter also casts a gaze towards the horizon of recent developments and ongoing research in the realm of the glue ear. Emerging treatments, innovative surgical techniques, and advanced hearing technologies paint a promising picture of the future. It is a future where the confluence of innovation, medical advancement, and deeper understanding holds the promise of enhanced quality of life for those affected by glue ear.

This journey through the medical treatments of the glue ear is not just about the interventions themselves. It is about offering hope, clarity, and pathways to better hearing and overall well-being. It is a testament to the remarkable progress and relentless pursuit of solutions in the world of otolaryngology.

Home Care and Lifestyle Changes

In the intricate dance of managing the glue ear, the steps taken at home and the rhythm of daily lifestyle choices play an integral role. This chapter is a journey through the various home care strategies and lifestyle adaptations that can effectively complement medical treatments, creating a symphony of holistic care.

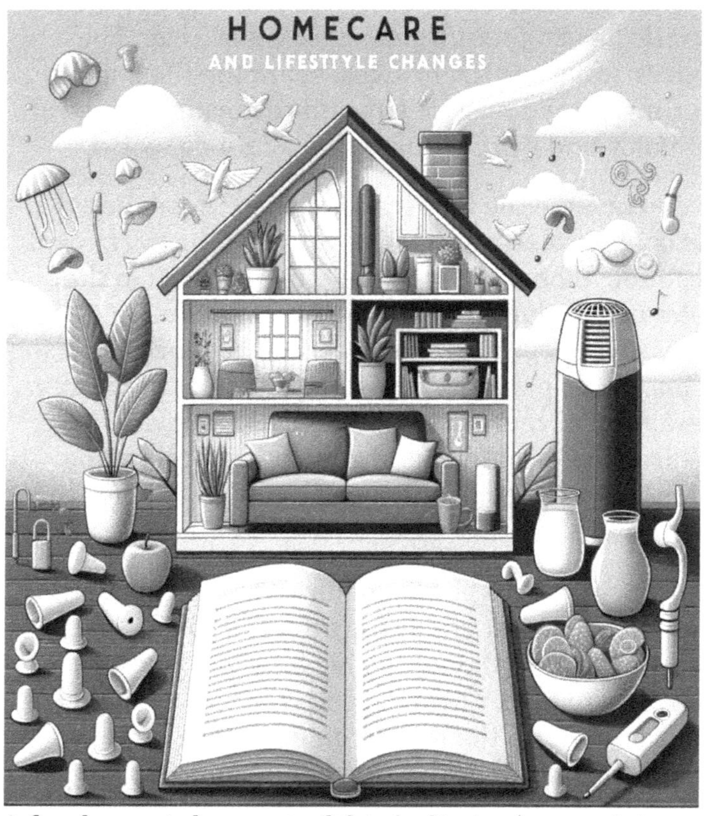

A fundamental aspect of this holistic approach is ear hygiene. Simple yet effective practices like keeping the ears dry can have a profound impact. This is important during activities such as bathing or swimming, where the ears are more exposed to water. The judicious use of earplugs or specially designed ear drops can block situations where contact with water is inevitable.

Another critical component in the home care of the glue ear is allergy management. For many, allergies are a key factor in the development and exacerbation of the glue ear. Keeping allergens at bay, therefore, can significantly alter the course of the condition. This might mean incorporating air purifiers into living spaces, opting for hypoallergenic bedding, or being vigilant about dietary choices to avoid food allergens.

People often downplay the role of diet and nutrition in managing the glue ear, yet it holds significant influence. A diet rich in anti-inflammatory foods can bolster the body's natural defenses against inflammation, indirectly contributing to the management of the glue ear. Similarly, staying well-hydrated is crucial, as adequate fluid intake is essential for the normal functioning of the mucous membranes, including those in the ears.

Beyond the physical strategies, this chapter also delves into the importance of emotional well-being. Dealing with a glue ear, especially when it's a long-standing companion, can be a taxing experience. Cultivating a supportive and understanding environment at home is crucial. Engaging in activities that reduce stress, fostering open and empathetic communication about the condition, and giving as much attention to emotional health as physical health are crucial in cultivating a supportive and understanding environment at home.

Empowerment is at the heart of this chapter–empowering you with the knowledge and tools to take a proactive role in managing the glue ear. It's about harmonizing the clinical aspects of care with the nuances of day-to-day living, weaving together a comprehensive approach to not just living with a glue ear but thriving despite it.

Living with Glue Ear

Early Life and Coping Strategies

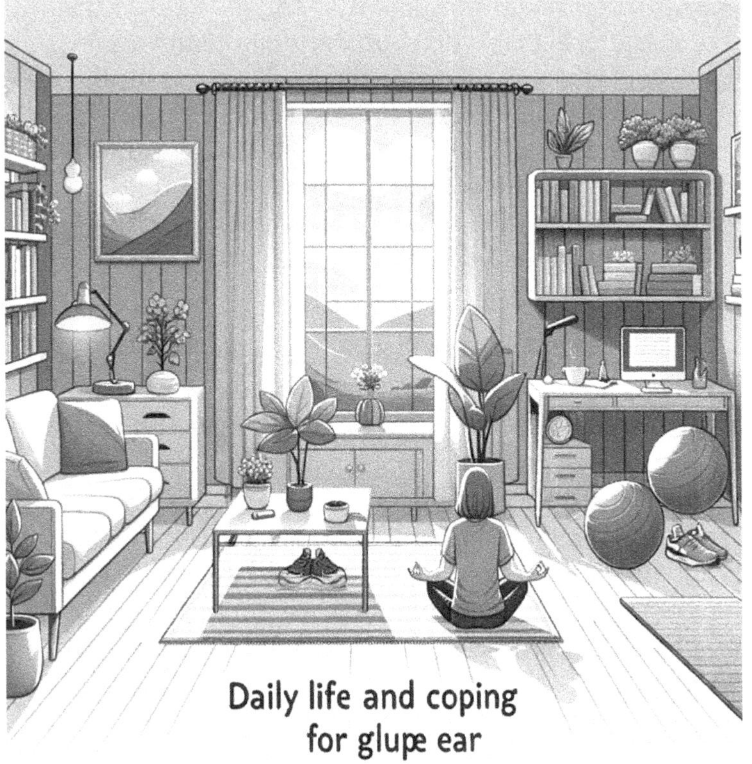

Navigating daily life with a glue ear can feel like walking through a world with an ever-shifting soundscape. This condition, known for its fluctuating symptoms, presents unique challenges that require resilience and adaptability. This chapter is a compass of practical coping strategies, aimed at improving the quality of life for those journeying with glue ear.

Effective Communication Techniques: One of the most significant challenges posed by the glue ear is the barrier it erects in communication. Mastering non-verbal cues such as facial expressions and gestures can be beneficial in bridging this gap. In a world where technology offers endless possibilities, tools like speech-to-text apps or hearing amplifiers can be transformative. They provide alternative avenues for staying connected and engaged in conversations.

Creating an Ear-Friendly Environment: The environments in which we live and work play a crucial role in managing the glue ear. One effective strategy is to minimize background noise, which can exacerbate hearing difficulties. Using sound-absorbing materials such as carpets, curtains, and soft furnishings can help create a more ear-friendly space. Being mindful of one's position during conversations — like facing the speaker and ensuring there's adequate lighting for visual cues — can enhance communication efficacy.

Stress Management and Relaxation: Stress can amplify the symptoms of the glue ear, making it imperative to integrate stress management and relaxation techniques into daily routines. Practices like mindfulness meditation and yoga not only offer a mental respite, but can also have positive effects on physical well-being. Engaging in hobbies or activities that bring joy and relaxation can also be a powerful tool in the stress management arsenal.

Physical Exercise: Regular physical activity is a cornerstone of overall health and can also contribute to ear health. Exercise enhances blood circulation, which is beneficial for all body functions, including those of the ear. Low-impact activities like walking or swimming (while using ear protection) are excellent options for maintaining fitness without putting undue stress on the ears.

Staying Informed and Proactive: In the ever-evolving landscape of healthcare, staying informed about the latest research and developments in the glue's treatment ear is empowering. It enables individuals to make well-informed decisions about their health and treatment options. Regular consultations with healthcare professionals are crucial as they provide opportunities for monitoring the condition and adapting treatment plans as necessary.

This chapter equips individuals with a glue ear with the tools and knowledge to navigate their daily lives more effectively. By implementing these strategies, one can not only cope with the challenges posed by the glue ear but also enhance their overall quality of life.

Support and Resources

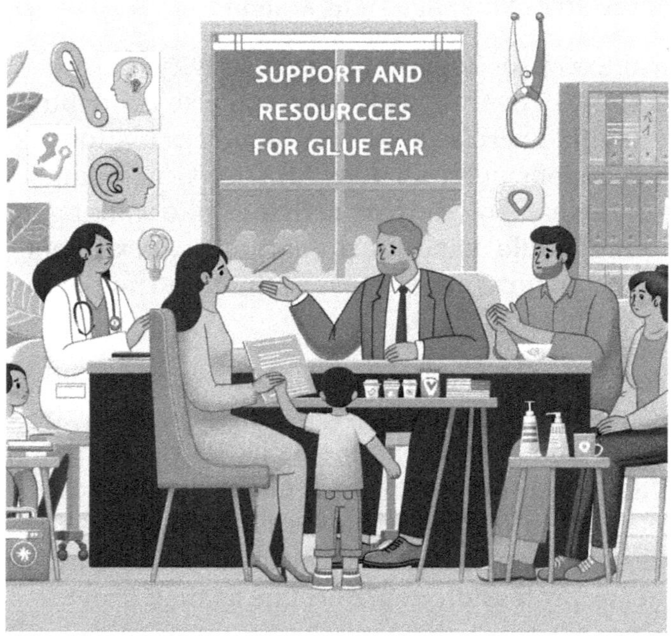

The journey with a glue ear, while personal, need not be a solitary one. This chapter focuses on the wealth of support and resources available, highlighting how tapping into these can make the journey less daunting and more manageable.

Professional Healthcare Support: Building a strong relationship with healthcare providers, such as audiologists, ENT specialists, and primary care physicians, is crucial. They can offer personalized advice, up-to-date treatments, and ongoing support.

Community and Online Support Groups: Joining support groups, either or online, can provide a platform to share experiences, tips, and receive emotional support from others who understand the challenges of living with a glue ear.

Educational Resources and Advocacy: Accessing reliable educational materials from reputable sources can provide valuable information about the glue ear. Advocacy groups can offer guidance on navigating healthcare systems and accessing necessary accommodations, especially in educational or workplace settings.

Family and Friends: Engaging with family and friends about the challenges of glue ear can help build a supportive home environment. Open communication about one's needs and how others can assist can strengthen relationships and improve daily interactions.

Using Assistive Technologies: There are many technological aids available, from specialized hearing devices to apps designed for those with hearing impairments. Exploring these options can improve communication and independence.

By embracing these strategies and resources, individuals with a glue ear can forge a path that not only navigates the challenges but also enhances their overall quality of life. This chapter aims to provide a roadmap for that journey, filled with support, understanding, and empowerment.

Chapter 4: Preventing Glue Ear

Preventing Glue Ear

While the glue ear can be a complex condition to manage, its prevention lies in the realm of possibility and practicality. This chapter sheds light on actionable strategies and tips to reduce the risk of developing the glue ear, emphasizing the power of proactive health measures.

Ear Hygiene and care: One of the simplest yet most effective preventive measures is maintaining good ear hygiene. This includes avoiding inserting objects into the ears, which can lead to injuries or infections. Keeping ears dry and clean, especially after swimming or bathing, can also play a crucial role in preventing glue ear.

Allergy Management: For those prone to allergies, managing these sensitivities can reduce the risk of glue ear. This may involve avoiding known allergens, using appropriate allergy medications, and maintaining a clean environment to minimize exposure to allergens like dust and pollen.

Healthy Lifestyle Choices: A healthy lifestyle that includes a balanced diet, regular exercise, and adequate hydration contributes to overall health and can aid in preventing glue ear. A diet rich in vitamins and minerals supports the immune system, while staying hydrated helps maintain the normal function of mucous membranes.

Avoiding Tobacco Smoke: Exposure to tobacco smoke, whether or through secondhand smoke, can increase the risk of glue ear. Avoiding smoking and minimizing exposure to smoke can be a significant step in prevention.

Regular Health Check-ups: Regular visits to healthcare providers, including ENT specialists, can help in early detection and management of any ear-related issues, preventing developing the glue ear.

Raising Awareness

Awareness and education about glue ear are pivotal in demystifying this common condition. This chapter focuses on spreading knowledge about the glue ear, aiming to bring it into the broader conversation about health and well-being.

Community Education: Educating the community about the glue ear, its symptoms, and its impact can foster a supportive environment. This can involve organizing or taking part in health talks, workshops, and information sessions in schools, workplaces, and community centers.

Role of Healthcare Professionals: Healthcare professionals play a vital role in raising awareness of the glue ear. This includes providing patients and their families with comprehensive information and advocating for greater awareness in the medical community health initiatives.

Using Media and Technology: Leveraging various media platforms, including social media, websites, and blogs, can help spread accurate information about the glue ear. Sharing personal stories, expert opinions, and educational content can reach a wide audience, increasing general understanding and empathy.

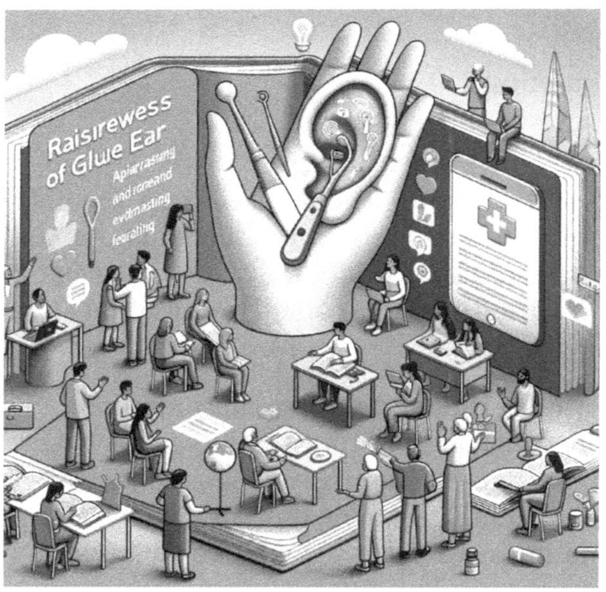

Collaboration with organizations: Collaborating with health organizations, advocacy groups, and educational institutions can amplify the message about the glue ear. These partnerships can cause more extensive outreach programs, research initiatives, and policy advocacy.

Empowerment through Knowledge:, raising awareness about glue ear empowers individuals to seek timely medical advice, support others in their community, and advocate for better health resources and policies.

By embracing both preventive measures and pursuing increased awareness, we can create a more informed and healthier society, where we understand, manage, and prevent glue ear.

Conclusion

As we draw the curtains on our exploration of the glue ear, it's essential to reflect on the key insights and wisdom gathered along this journey. Glue ear, a condition as common as it is complex, affects individuals across all ages, each facing unique challenges and experiences. Yet, the thread that weaves through every chapter of this narrative is the power of understanding and proactive health management.

From the intricacies of symptoms and diagnosis in various age groups to the comprehensive approaches to treatment and management, we've traversed a landscape rich in information and guidance. Prizing medical interventions, be they antibiotics, ear tubes, or advanced surgical options, stands as a testament to the advancements in healthcare and the hope they offer. significant is the role of home care and lifestyle changes, highlighting how daily choices and practices can influence our health journey.

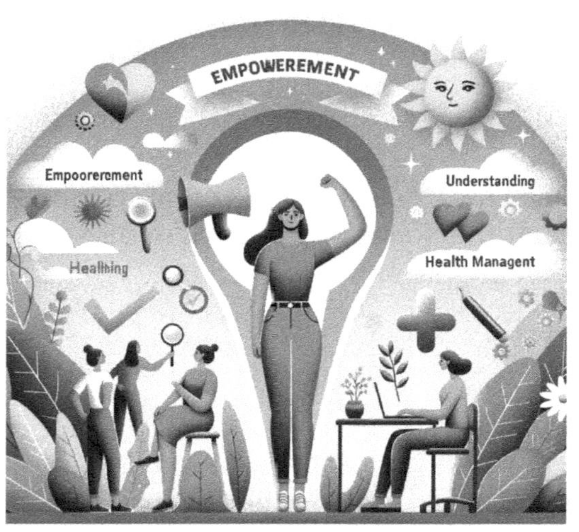

Prevention and awareness have emerged as crucial allies in this endeavor. By adopting preventive measures like maintaining ear hygiene, managing allergies, and leading a healthy lifestyle, we can reduce the risk of developing the glue ear. Raising awareness empowers communities, breaks down stigmas, and fosters an environment where the glue ear is not just understood but managed.

In concluding, the message is simple: proactive health management, combined with a deep understanding of glue ear, can enhance the quality of life for those affected. It's a call to action for individuals, healthcare professionals, and communities alike to embrace the knowledge, engage in open conversations, and advocate for better health practices. As we close this chapter, let's carry forward the spirit of empowerment and vigilance, ensuring that support, understanding, and resilience marks the journey with a glue ear.

Chapter 5: Glue Ear Alternatives

Exploring different avenues for treating the glue ear can be a revelation. Often, conventional methods like surgery or standard medication might not be everyone's cup of tea, especially for those who prefer a gentler approach. Let's dive into some intriguing alternatives that might just do the trick.

1. The Natural Approach to Tackling Glue Ear

Unveiling Nature's Remedies for Glue Ear

In the grand saga of managing a glue ear, a condition that can be as sticky as its name suggests, we often overlook nature's own medicine cabinet. This chapter delves into the world of natural remedies, offering a green thumb's guide to easing the discomfort and muffled hearing caused by this pesky ear condition.

Glue Ear: The Sticky Culprit

Picture your ear as a tiny concert hall, now filled with an unwanted, gooey guest–fluid. Glue ear is like an uninvited party crasher, clogging up the Eustachian tube, which keeps the middle ear's air-flowing and sound-waves bouncing. The result? Muffled tunes and a lot of discomfort, especially for the little ones.

Herbal Heroes: Nature's Line-up Against Glue Ear

In the lush, vibrant world of herbal remedies, several standout stars offer a symphony of relief:

Goldenseal: Nature's Antibacterial Maestro

- Imagine a plant with roots deep in Native American medicine, wielding a compound named berberine like a conductor's baton. It orchestrates a powerful antibacterial melody, making it a prime candidate to take on ear infections.

Chamomile: The Soothing Soprano

- Known for its calming lullabies and anti-inflammatory notes, chamomile tea, when cooled and used as ear drops, can soothe the inflamed ear passages like a gentle serenade.

Garlic: The Pungent Protector

- Beyond its role in the kitchen, garlic emerges as a natural antibiotic and antifungal virtuoso. A few drops of warm garlic oil in the ear work like a covert agent, battling the infection.

Echinacea: The Immune System's Cheerleader

- This herb takes on the role of boosting the body's immune choir, helping it hit the high notes in fighting off infections. Whether in tea or supplement form, it's a holistic encore for overall ear health.

The Art of Using Herbal Remedies: A Responsible Approach

Even nature's remedies require a thoughtful, informed approach. Always conduct a pre-show allergy test, consult with a healthcare maestro before starting any new herbal protocol, and seek the highest quality, organic ingredients for the best performance.

A Step-by-Step Guide to Harmonizing Ear Health

Incorporating these herbal remedies into your daily routine can be as simple and harmonious as a well-practiced musical scale:

- Goldenseal: Blend the powder with warm water to create a soothing ear drop concerto.
- Chamomile: Let the tea cool down and use it as a gentle, calming ear drop.
- Garlic Oil: Warm the oil for a soothing, infection-fighting melody in the ear.

The Science Behind the Remedies: More Than Just Folklore

These herbal remedies are not mere folklore; the symphony of science backs them. Their antibacterial and anti-inflammatory properties have been shown to play a significant role in combating the symptoms of the glue ear.

Success Stories: Real-life Testimonials

Many anecdotes sing the praises of these natural remedies. From parents witnessing the dramatic improvement in their children to adults finding solace in these herbal tunes, the success stories are as inspiring as they are validating.

Conclusion: Embracing Nature's Symphony

In conclusion, while the modern medical orchestra offers various solutions for the glue ear, the gentle yet potent power of natural remedies deserves a standing ovation. With their ability to manage symptoms and often with fewer side effects, these herbal remedies are a testament to the healing melodies of Mother Nature.

As we close this chapter, let's remember the key is responsible use and harmonizing these natural solutions with professional advice. Whether it's Goldenseal's antibacterial command, Chamomile's soothing lullaby, Garlic's hidden strength, or Echinacea's immune-boosting anthem, nature has provided us with a diverse and powerful ensemble to support our journey towards ear health. So, if you battle the discomfort of the glue ear, consider tuning into the healing rhythms of these natural remedies. 🌱🎶

2. Embracing Innovative Solutions for Glue Ear

The Otovent Nasal Balloon: A Whimsical Yet Effective Remedy

In the world of ear health, when battling the clingy foe known as the glue ear, innovation takes center stage with the Otovent Nasal Balloon. This section of our chapter whisks us into the effective realm of this simple, yet ingenious device.

Understanding Glue Ear: Setting the Stage

Before we get to the star of the show, let's set the scene. Glue ear, like a mischievous sprite, turns the middle ear into a pool of unwanted fluid. It's all thanks to a tiny but crucial part called the Eustachian tube, which, when blocked, becomes a bottleneck for trouble.

Meet the Otovent: A Hero in Disguise

Enter the Otovent, a nasal balloon that's like a magic wand in the world of glue ear. It's not a child's plaything;

The Magic Trick: How the Otovent Works

The Otovent's performance is a simple three-act play:

- Setup: The balloon, attached to a nozzle, is ready for its debut.
- Action: You block one nostril, insert the nozzle in the other, and blow. This inflates the balloon, and here's where the magic happens.
- Ta-day! The inflated balloon creates a gentle pressure, nudging the Eustachian tube open, allowing the fluid to drain like a curtain falling after a grand show.

Why It's Standing Ovation-Worthy

- Simplicity: It's non-invasive, requiring just a balloon and a breath.
- Child-Friendly: Even younglings, as tender as three years old, can join in.
- Effectiveness: Backed by studies, it's proven to be a reliable sidekick in combating the glue ear.

The Science Behind the Balloon: A Pressure Play

It's all about the pressure. The act of inflating the balloon creates a pressure change, a gentle nudge that reminds the Eustachian tube of its duties. It's like coaxing a shy performer onto the stage, restoring balance and harmony to the middle ear.

Otovent in Action: A Step-by-Step Guide

- Prepare the Stage: Attach the balloon.
- Position: Insert the nozzle into one nostril.
- The Mann Act: Inflate the balloon with a gentle blow.
- Encore: Repeat the routine thrice daily, as recommended.

Safety Curtain: Tips for a Smooth Performance

- Gentle Approach: Think of it as a feather-light touch, not a gusty wind.
- Cleanliness: Keep the nozzle pristine, like a polished stage.
- Doctor's Nod: Always get a thumbs-up from your healthcare maestro.

Success Stories: Applause from the Audience

From children rediscovering the joy of clear hearing to adults bidding farewell to that underwater echo, the Otovent has a fanbase singing its praises.

FAQs: Curious Minds Want to Know

- Timeframe for Results: A few weeks of regular use can bring the curtain up on improvements.
- Age No Bar: Suitable for both young and mature audiences alike.
- A Long-term Fix? While it offers a standing ovation-worthy performance, consulting a healthcare professional for an encore strategy is wise.

Conclusion: A Breath of Fresh Air in Ear Health

To wrap up this act, the Otovent Nasal Balloon is like a fresh breeze in the world of glue ear management. Simple, safe, and with a sprinkle of whimsy, it's a solution that can turn the tides in the battle against this clingy ailment. For those seeking a non-invasive route to clearer ears and brighter days, this little balloon might just be the ticket to a happy, healthier ear-venture.

3. Deciphering Glue Ear with Advanced Diagnostic Tools

Pneumatic Otoscopy and Tympanometry: Illuminating the Depths of Glue Ear

In our quest to unravel the mysteries of the glue ear, we embark on a journey with two technological allies: Pneumatic Otoscopy and tympanometry. This section of our chapter shines a light on how these tools not only diagnose but also contribute to managing the glue ear.

Glue Ear Unveiled: A Fluid Dilemma

To set the stage, let's revisit the glue ear. Picture your ear as a cozy room, with the Eustachian tube serving as a door that swings open to regulate air and drain fluid. Now imagine this door gets stuck–the result is a build-up of fluid, leading to muffled hearing. This is the essence of the glue ear.

Pneumatic Otoscopy: Peering into the Ear's Secrets

Pneumatic Otoscopy may sound like a gadget from a future era, but it's a straightforward tool that provides a window into the ear's inner workings.

- What It Does: It employs a pneumatic otoscope to examine the eardrum, with gentle puffs of air revealing the eardrum's reaction.
- Why It's Crucial: It detects fluid behind the eardrum and assesses the eardrum's mobility, both key factors in identifying glue ear.

Tympanometry: The Ear's Pressure Gauge

Tympanometry, though it sounds complex, is a fascinating tool that measures the eardrum's response to air pressure variations.

- Its Function: It involves a device that alters air pressure in the ear, causing the eardrum to vibrate. Then, the device measures these vibrations.
- Its Role in Glue Ear: It excels in identifying fluid in the middle ear and evaluating the Eustachian tube's function.

A Deep Dive: The Procedures Explained

Both Pneumatic Otoscopy and tympanometry are non-invasive, pain-free, and swift, making them suitable for all ages.

- Pneumatic Otoscopy: The process involves sitting still while the doctor places the otoscope in your ear and observes the eardrum's response to air puffs.
- Tympanometry: Involves inserting a soft tip into the ear, changing the ear's pressure, and recording the eardrum's reaction.

Interpreting the Results: A Guide to Ear Health

These tests provide valuable insights:

- Pneumatic Otoscopy Findings: Normal movement shows a fluid-free middle ear, while restricted movement suggests fluid build-up.
- Tympanometry Data: A Type A Curve signals normality, while Type B or C may show fluid or Eustachian tube issues.

Ensuring Comfort and Safety

We design these tests with safety and minimal discomfort in mind. A slight pressure sensation is normal during tympanometry but should not cause pain.

Post-Test Protocol

- Aftermath:, there are no side effects post-test.
- Results Discussion: Your doctor will decode the findings and discuss their implications.

FAQs: Addressing Your Concerns

- Child-Friendly?: Yes, they are both child-friendly and tolerated well by young patients.
- Duration: Each test takes just a few minutes.
- Necessity for diagnosis: They are among the most reliable tools for diagnosing glue ear.

Conclusion: Charting a Path to Better Ear Health

In summary, Pneumatic Otoscopy and tympanometry are indispensable in the battle against glue ear. They offer a detailed snapshot of middle ear health, essential for informed treatment decisions. Whether you're navigating this as a parent or as an individual, these tests are crucial steps towards improved ear health.

Understanding your condition is the cornerstone of effective treatment. By embracing these diagnostic technologies, you're not just gaining insight into your ear's condition; you're steering your health journey towards a brighter, clearer future. ✳ ⬤ 🔍

Probiotics: Harnessing Good Bacteria in the Fight Against Glue Ear

In the intricate world of ear health, and in the glue ear, the role of probiotics emerges as a surprising yet promising ally. This section of our chapter delves into how these microscopic warriors can help to manage the glue ear.

Glue Ear: The Persistent Blockage

To understand the potential of probiotics, let's first revisit the glue ear. Imagine your ear feels like it's underwater, making hearing a Herculean task. This condition arises from the build-up of fluid in the middle ear, a situation that can distress for children.

Probiotics: The Benevolent Microorganisms

Probiotics are live microorganisms that benefit our health, known for their positive impact on the digestive system. Interestingly, their influence extends to areas including the ear and throat.

The Probiotic-Glue Ear Nexus

- Microbial Balance: Probiotics help maintain a healthy bacterial environment in the ear and throat.

- Immune Enhancement: They play a crucial role in bolstering the immune system, a key defense against the onset of glue ear.

Probiotic Varieties for Ear Health

Different probiotics offer various benefits, but for ear health, certain strains stand out:

- Lactobacillus: found in yogurt and fermented foods.
- Bifidobacterium: present in dairy products.

Mechanics of Probiotics Against Glue Ear

The intrigue lies in how probiotics maintain a bacterial balance in the ear and throat, preventing conditions conducive to fluid accumulation.

The Science Unveiled

- Infection Combat: Strengthening the immune system, probiotics reduce infection risks that can lead to the glue ear.
- Bacterial Harmony: They are essential in sustaining a healthy bacterial equilibrium, critical for ear health.

Incorporating Probiotics for Glue Ear

Considering probiotics for glue ear management involves:

- Professional Consultation: Begin with advice from a healthcare provider.

- Strain Selection: Opt for probiotics known for their benefits in ear health.

Integrating Probiotics into Your Diet

- Yogurt: A tasty, probiotic-rich option.
- Supplements: An alternative for those who avoid dairy.

Safety and Potential Side Effects

While safe, it's important to be aware of:

- Digestive Reactions: Some may experience bloating or gas.
- Allergic Concerns: Rare but noteworthy.

Success Stories: Testimonials of Relief

Many individuals, from children to adults, have reported improvements in ear health following probiotic use, offering hope and evidence of their efficacy.

FAQs: Addressing Common Queries

- The timeframe for results: Patients often notice improvements within weeks, but this can vary.
- Probiotics act as a cure by aiding in symptom management and prevention.

Conclusion: Probiotics as a Gentle Force in Ear Health

In summary, probiotics, while not associated with ear health, present a natural and gentle method for managing the glue ear. They fortify the immune system and ensure a healthy bacterial balance, which can be critical in preventing and managing the glue ear.

It's important to tailor the approach to each individual's needs, and consulting a healthcare provider is crucial. However, for many, probiotics have emerged as a valuable component of their ear health strategy, offering a beacon of hope and comfort in the struggle against the glue ear. Consider probiotics as your tiny, yet formidable allies in the journey towards maintaining ear health.

5. Pneumatic Otoscopy and Tympanometry: Diagnostics Turned Treatment Pneumatic Otoscopy and Tympanometry: Unlocking the Mysteries of Glue Ear

Navigating the world of ear health can sometimes feel like trying to solve a complex puzzle. For those struggling with the glue ear, two key pieces of this puzzle are Pneumatic Otoscopy and tympanometry. Let's explore how these innovative tools not only diagnose but also contribute to treating the glue ear.

Understanding Glue Ear: A Sticky Challenge

Before we delve into these diagnostic tools, let's touch base on what glue ear is. Imagine your ear as a small room with a door that stays open to let air in and out.

This door is your Eustachian tube. Now, what if this door gets stuck? Fluid accumulates, and hearing becomes muffled. That's a glue ear for you.

Pneumatic Otoscopy: A Window to Your Ear

Pneumatic Otoscopy might sound like something out of a sci-fi movie, but it's a simple and insightful way to look inside the ear.

What Is Pneumatic Otoscopy?

- Definition: It's a procedure where a doctor uses a special tool called a pneumatic otoscope to examine your ear, especially the eardrum.
- How It Works: puffing air into the ear causes the eardrum to move. Movement (or lack of it) gives clues about what's happening inside.

Why It Matters for Glue Ear?

- Detects Fluid: This tool can show if there's fluid behind the eardrum, a common issue with a glue ear.
- Assesses Eardrum Mobility: It helps to see how well the eardrum can move, which is crucial for hearing.

Tympanometry: Measuring Ear Health

Tympanometry sounds even more technical, but it's just as fascinating and useful.

Understanding Tympanometry

- What It Is: Tympanometry is a test that measures how the eardrum responds to changes in air pressure.
- We place a device in the ear to change the air pressure and make the eardrum vibrate. We measure this vibration afterwards.Its Role in Glue Ear Management
- Identifies Fluid Buildup: Tympanometry can detect fluid in the middle ear, even when it's not infected.
- Evaluates Eustachian Tube Function: It gives a clear picture of how well the Eustachian tube is working, which is often the root problem in the glue ear.

A Closer Look: The Procedure Explained

Both Pneumatic Otoscopy and tympanometry are non-invasive, painless, and quick, making them ideal for all ages.

Pneumatic Otoscopy Step-by-Step

- Preparation: Sit still and relax. The doctor will explain each step.
- During the examination, the doctor places the otoscope in your ear and releases a small puff of air.
- Observation: The doctor watches how your eardrum moves in response to the air.

Tympanometry in Action

- During the setup, the technician places a soft tip attached to the tympano meter in your ear.
- Pressure Changes: The machine changes the pressure in your ear and produces a tone.
- Recording: The device records the eardrum's response to these changes.

Interpreting the Results: What Do They Mean?

The results from these tests can tell your doctor a lot about your ear health.

Decoding Pneumatic Otoscopy

- Normal Movement: shows that the middle ear is likely free of fluid.
- Restricted Movement: Could point to fluid buildup, suggesting glue ear.

Understanding Tympanometry Data

- Type A Curve: Normal pressure and mobility.
- Type B or C Curve: shows issues like fluid buildup or Eustachian tube dysfunction.

Safety and Comfort: Ensuring a Smooth Experience

These tests are safe, with minimal discomfort. It's normal to feel a bit of pressure during tympanometry, but it shouldn't be painful.

After the Test

- No Side Effects: Most people feel fine after these tests.

- Discuss Results: Your doctor will explain what the findings mean for your ear health.

FAQs: Answering Your Burning Questions

- Q: Can we perform these tests on children?
- A:! They are safe and well-tolerated by kids.
- Q: How long do the tests take?
- A: They're quick–just a few minutes each.
- Q: Do I need these tests for diagnosing glue ear?
- A: They are among the best tools for diagnosing glue ear.

Conclusion: Empowering Your Ear Health Journey

In conclusion, Pneumatic Otoscopy and tympanometry are invaluable tools in the fight against glue ear. They provide detailed insights into the health of your middle ear and are crucial for making informed decisions about treatment. Whether you're a concerned parent or an adult troubled by persistent ear issues, these tests can be a key step toward better ear health.

Remember, understanding your condition is the first step in addressing it. By embracing these diagnostic tools, you're not just getting a clearer picture of what's happening in your ear; you're taking an active role in your health care journey. So, next time you visit your doctor for ear troubles, you'll know what these tests are all about and how they can help you.

Conclusion: Navigating the Maze of Glue Ear Treatments

When tackling glue ear, a variety of treatments are available, each offering unique benefits. From the natural healing of herbs and probiotics to the innovative technology of Otovent nasal balloons and autoinflation devices, options abound. Pneumatic otoscopy and tympanometry also provide critical diagnostic insights, aiding in effective management.

It's essential to remember that every health journey is personal, and what works for one may not work for another. Exploring resources like CureHacks for natural remedies or consulting healthcare professionals about the latest devices can guide you in making informed choices. Ultimately, each treatment path opens a new avenue for managing glue ear, offering hope and relief to many. With the right information and guidance, you can make empowered decisions about your health and well-being, harnessing a blend of nature's wisdom and modern medical advances.

Bonus Chapter 1: 80s?

Although focus in on 80's in this chapter, it is for anyone of any age who may also have chronic issues.

Glue ear, known as otitis media with effusion (OME), occurs when fluid, often thick and sticky, builds up inside the middle ear without a clear sign of infection. This fluid weighs down the eardrum and tiny bones in the middle ear, causing hearing loss, ear fullness, and other symptoms. While glue ear is very common in younger children, few people realize seniors over 80 can also be impacted by it.

Glue ear happens after a cold or ear infection, when the tubes connecting that connect the ears and throat get blocked and prevent fluid from draining. While children often "grow out of" the condition as their tubes widen, older adults have less ability to recover from persistent fluid, build up and restore drainage on their own. In fact, age-related changes to our Eustachian tubes and immunity make seniors especially vulnerable.

Unfortunately, many elderly patients (and even some physicians) assume hearing loss and related ear issues are an inevitable part of aging. But glue ear is often reversible - and allowing it to become chronic can increase the chances of long-term damage, substantial hearing impairment, balance problems that increase fall risk, and depression/social isolation. Being attuned to the signs of glue ear and discussing symptoms with doctors is key for the 80+ crowd.

The good news is, we have effective tools to catch glue ear early and treat it - including patient-friendly medical therapy and minor ear drainage procedures done under local anesthetic on an outpatient basis. By better understanding glue ear causes, risks factors, and solutions, over 80s can protect their ears and hearing for years to come.

Glue ear can be tricky to identify, especially in seniors whose hearing seems to get worse bit by bit, anyway. The most common symptom of the glue ear is mild or worsening hearing loss, often in both ears. Sound may seem softer or more muffled than normal. You might struggle to understand people's speech, or need to turn up the TV volume higher than usual. Other symptoms include:

- A feeling that your ears are full or clogged

- Ringing in your ears (tinnitus)

- Poor balance, dizziness, or unsteadiness

Now, the tricky thing is that these symptoms can seem to come and go. Sometimes the stickiness drains and hearing returns closer to normal, while at other times is it quite dampened. This fluctuating nature makes glue ear harder to recognize.

Also, since many elderly people have age-related hearing loss, you may not even pick up on extra changes from the glue ear. Or you might chalk it up to "getting older" rather than a true inflammation issue that warrants medical treatment. This makes checking your hearing ability important.

If you suspect you might have a glue ear, see your doctor. They will examine inside the ear with an instrument called an otoscope, looking for fluid. Doctors perform a test called tympanometry to check for problems with the flexibility of the eardrum. You may also get a standard hearing exam to map out the type and hearing loss. These tests together can confirm if the glue ear is present. Getting the right diagnosis is the critical first step towards regaining your best possible hearing ability over 80.

Why Glue Ear is More Common in Those Over 80

To understand why seniors are vulnerable to glue ear, you first need to know how it develops. Glue ear occurs after having a cold, sinus infection, allergy flare-up, or other respiratory illness. This inflammation and mucus production causes swelling in the back of the nose and throat, including the area called the nasopharynx.

Within this area sit the Eustachian tubes - small channels running from the middle ear space down to the throat. These tubes help regulate air pressure and drain fluid from the ears to the back of the nose and throat. However, if our Eustachian tubes get blocked or bogged down by swelling, that fluid can get stuck in the ear and accumulate.

As we age, several natural changes occur that make this process more likely. The cartilage support around our Eustachian tubes weakens, causing them to be more floppy and collapse more easily. Our immune systems also slow down, making respiratory illnesses and infections harder to recover from. Conditions like acid reflux, with stomach contents backing up towards the ears, become more common too.

On top of that, many elderly people have chronic issues like sinusitis, adenoid issues, or allergies that can cause persistent inflammation and fluid build-up. Certain medications are another risk factor - especially blood pressure treatments, diuretics, arthritis drugs, and even OTC antihistamines or decongestants sometimes.

With multiple age-related physical changes and health conditions jeopardizing our Eustachian tubes and drainage, it is no wonder seniors are prone to developing a stubborn glue ear. Staying vigilant to ear symptoms and consulting your doctor for diagnosis and treatment is key, as the problem resolves without intervention after age 80. Getting ahead of glue ear protects seniors against losing more precious hearing.

The Lasting Harm Glue Ear Can Cause

Left unchecked over time, the glue ear can cause more than just temporary hearing loss for the elderly. The inflammation and fluid prevent the proper transmission of sound through the middle ear, which can "shut down" parts of the inner ear and auditory nerve pathways.

As an analogy, think of how a cast immobilizing a broken bone for too long causes stiffness or muscle wasting. Lack of proper stimulation to the hearing mechanisms allows the structures and pathways to degrade. In medical terms, the hair cells and nerves can atrophy.

Over time, this makes hearing loss chronic rather than temporary. More severely impaired hearing from the glue ear also makes tinnitus (ringing ears) or balance issues more likely. The damage also stacks on top of natural age-related hearing decline most people develop.

Chronic hearing impairment puts seniors at risk for other medical problems. Struggling to communicate leads many older adults to withdraw and isolate. This raises risks for depression, cognitive decline, and dementia according to research. Untreated glue ear also causes stress for caregivers trying to communicate with a senior with hearing loss.

There are also links between poor hearing and problems with memory, mobility, and falling - all critical issues for the elderly. The bottom line is listening to symptoms and intervening with glue ear diagnosis and management prevents far more extensive consequences than just frustrating muffled hearing episodes now and then. Safeguarding hearing health remains a priority well into later life.

The good news when glue ear strikes in your later years is that effective treatments options exist without extensive surgery or medications that put elderly patients at higher risk. Doctors tailor glue ear management approaches based both on the severity of symptoms and health/medication considerations more common with advanced age.

Mild glue ear often first gets "watched" for improvement over a few weeks. Staying well hydrated, using saline nasal sprays, or taking an oral decongestant may help fluid drain. Be aware common OTC antihistamine decongestants like diphenhydramine often cause confusion or urinary retention in seniors though.

If glue ear persists and causes hearing problems, physicians may prescribe a steroid nasal spray or even a brief regimen of oral steroids. Stronger prescription decongestant drops with less anticholinergic effects are another option. Always consult your doctor before starting any new medication over 80 though, even OTC ones.

For severe or chronic glue ear in seniors not responsive to other treatments, ear tube surgery remains the most definitive option. This minor procedure places tiny tubes to ventilate the middle ear space and facilitate drainage. It's done under local anesthesia. After a brief recovery, tubes often restore hearing to near normal until they fall out on their own in 6 months.

Working with your doctors helps determine the right glue ear treatment plan for your individual health history and symptoms. Don't just assume hearing changes must be permanent or untreatable because of age. Advocate for your ear health by speaking up about symptoms early and giving medical therapies a try before permanent damage sets in.

Reducing Your Glue Ear Risks Over 80

While some age-related physical changes raise glue, ear risks are unavoidable, seniors can still take proactive steps to minimize chances of developing this troublesome condition. Prevention centers on avoiding the respiratory illnesses and inflammation that often trigger glue ear.

It starts with infection control basics like washing hands, avoiding contact with sick people, and getting your annual flu shot. Treating nasal allergies or sinus irritations when they flare up is wise too. Quitting smoking and improving air quality at home also helps reduce ear inflammation risks.

Some over-the-counter options exist to help relieve congestion problems that contribute to glue ear episodes. Saline nasal rinses and sprays help thin out sticky nasal secretions and open Eustachian tube openings. Staying well hydrated also thins out mucus.

Over 80s should use OTC nasal decongestants because of higher risk of side effects like fast heart rate, confusion, dizziness and falling. But prescription nasal steroid sprays, when taken and monitored by a doctor, are safe and quite effective for chronic nasal congestion.

At home, be alert to any hearing, ear fullness, or balance changes after you've had a cold or allergy flare up. Follow up with your physician if symptoms don't resolve after a week or two. The sooner you receive a diagnosis and treatment plan tailored to your health status, the better your outcome with a glue ear.

Protecting Your Hearing Health for Years to Come

Many people underestimate glue ear as a reversible condition in seniors, similar to other age-related health issues. Many people tolerate mild hearing loss or ear problems as an expected part of aging. However, a glue ear deserves attention since allowing it to become chronic can speed up senior hearing loss and balance issues leading to injury and social isolation.

The keys are understanding your personal risk factors, recognizing symptoms early, and consulting your doctor for diagnosis and treatment if ear troubles crop up after illnesses. By making lifestyle adjustments, prescribing suitable medications for individuals over 80, and performing minor ear procedures if necessary, healthcare professionals can often manage the glue ear.

While the glue ear may sound like a trivial childhood annoyance, it can impact quality of life for older adults in later years. Prioritizing ear health pays dividends through better communication, mobility, and independence. You owe it to yourself and loved ones to speak up about ear changes and explore solutions - good hearing and balance contribute so much to healthy, engaged aging.

Here's to staying connected and active, enjoying your golden years ahead!

Bonus Chapter 2: Grommets?

Picture yourself at 80, when life should be about enjoying the golden years, but instead, you're constantly battling hearing loss, feeling isolated in conversations, and dealing with recurring ear discomfort. Many seniors live with a condition called glue ear, where fluid build-up in the middle ear causes hearing loss and frequent infections. It's more than just a medical problem.o ask for repetitions or miss out on the soft whispers of a grandchild. In this situation, finding a solution becomes imperative.

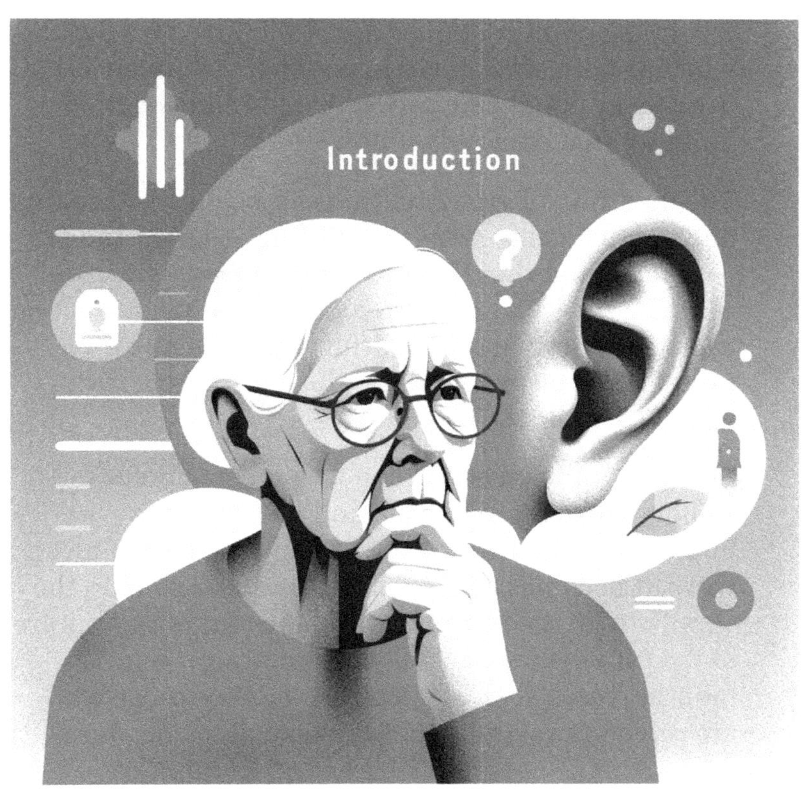

Understanding Grommet Tubes

Grommet tubes, also called tympanostomy tubes, provide hope for seniors dealing with glue ear. These small cylinders are inserted into the eardrum, creating a pathway for air and fluid flow. This device, which is both simple and ingenious, can enhance hearing by equalizing pressure and reducing fluid build-up that dampens sound.

The insertion of grommet tubes is a simple procedure done with local anesthesia, offering relief for those worried about the risks of general anesthesia in old age. The surgeon performs a myringotomy by making a small incision in the eardrum and inserting the tube.The surgeon completes the entire process in about 15 minutes.

Grommet tube insertion can be a turning point for seniors, improving hearing and reducing ear infections. When antibiotics or nasal steroids don't work, it becomes a valuable choice. Additionally, the simplicity of the procedure and the temporary nature of the tubes (they naturally dislodge after 6 to 12 months) make it an attractive option for those who are reluctant to undergo more invasive procedures.

However, it's crucial to recognize that although grommet tubes can revolutionize things, they don't work for everyone. It is essential to consult with an ENT specialist to determine if this path is suitable for your specific situation. Seniors like us must carefully weigh the benefits and risks of any medical procedure, considering our age and health.ubes often comes after weighing the potential benefits, which can be significant, especially for seniors like us. One of the most immediate and profound advantages is the improvement in hearing. By allowing the trapped fluid to drain and air to circulate in the middle ear, these tubes can restore hearing to a more normal level. This improvement is not just about being able to hear better; it's about reconnecting with our surroundings, engaging in conversations more confidently, and enjoying the sounds of life that we might have been missing out on.

Another major benefit is the reduction in ear infections. Chronic ear infections can be a painful and recurring problem for those with the glue ear, leading to discomfort and further hearing issues. Grommet tubes help prevent these infections by keeping the middle ear aerated and draining, reducing the risk of bacteria and viruses taking hold.

For seniors, the simplicity and safety of the procedure itself are significant pros. The insertion of grommet tubes is an invasive surgery, quick, and performed as an outpatient procedure. This means we can avoid the risks associated with more extensive surgeries and the longer recovery times that can be challenging for older adults.

Grommet tubes can be a relief for those who have found little success with other treatments like antibiotics or nasal sprays. They offer an alternative when traditional methods don't provide the needed relief, or when the side effects of medications become a concern.

Cons of Grommet Tubes

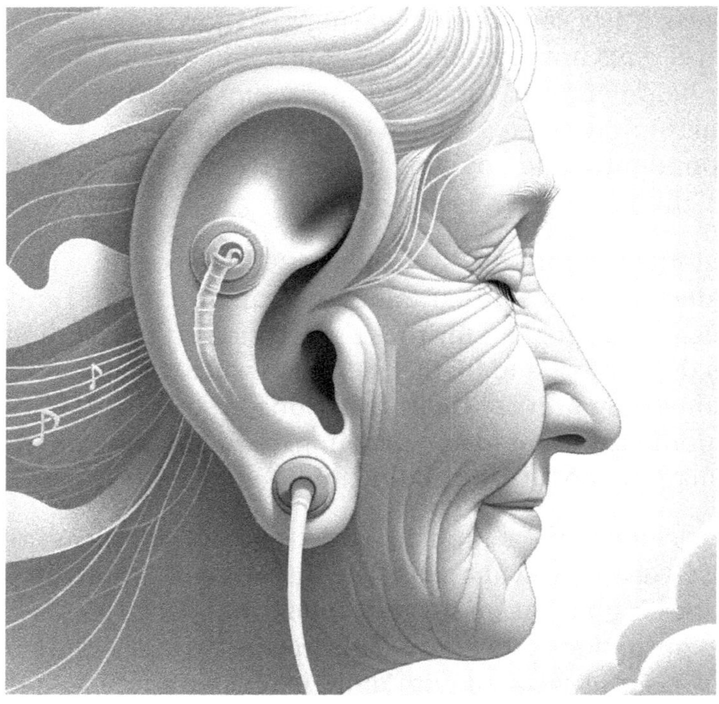

While the advantages of grommet tubes can be significant, it's important to consider their potential drawbacks, especially for seniors. One of the major concerns is the risk associated with any surgical procedure. Even though the insertion of grommet tubes is minimally invasive and safe, there are still risks of complications such as infection, bleeding, or reactions to anesthesia, albeit rare. This risk might be higher for seniors because of age-related factors and potential comorbidities.

Another issue to consider is the possibility of the tubes not functioning as intended.

Sometimes, the tubes might become blocked, fall out, or cannot improve hearing. There's also the risk of the tubes staying in place longer than necessary, which might require another procedure to remove them.

Scarring of the eardrum is a potential long-term complication. While this is rare, it's a concern to be aware of, as it can affect ear health and hearing. After placing the tubes, some individuals might require additional medical attention because of persistent drainage from the ear.

It should be mentioned that grommet tubes only alleviate glue ear symptoms, not the root cause. As a result, if the tubes are removed or fall out, fluid can build up once more, leading to the recurrence of the initial issues. Patients should consider the drawbacks and benefits, and consult with a healthcare professional when making this decision. Personalized advice can be given by the healthcare professional, taking into account individual health status and medical history.

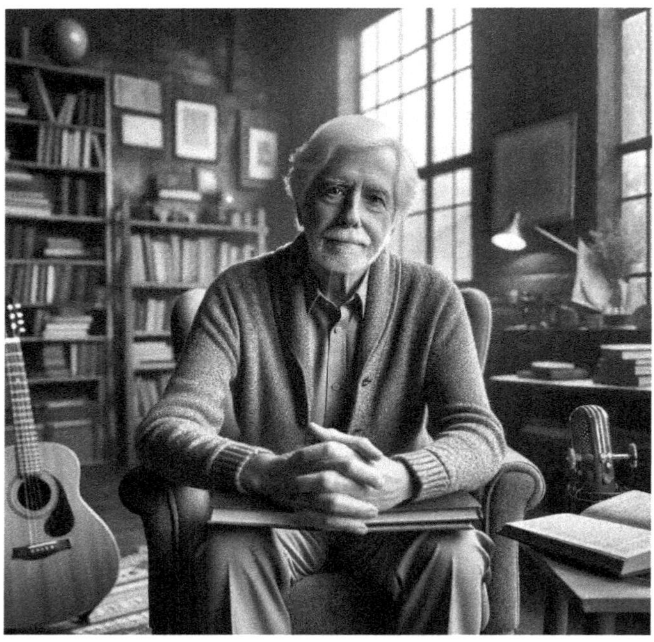

The insights from those who have had grommet tubes can be incredibly valuable., an 82-year-old retired teacher, who dealt with glue ear for several years. Despite attempting different therapies, his hearing continued to worsen, impacting his social interactions and overall well-being.

Following a detailed consultation with his ENT specialist, George decided to undergo the procedure for grommet tube insertion. The improvement in his hearing was astonishingly immediate. He compared it to a veil being removed, enabling him to have conversations without needing others to repeat themselves. His daily activities and interactions returned to normal with this positive change.

However, George's journey wasn't without its challenges. In the weeks after the procedure, he had a bit of discomfort and a small amount of ear discharge. Yet, George was able to resolve these issues through proper care and follow-up appointments. After approximately one year, the tubes came out and George's hearing continued to be better than before the procedure.

The story of George showcases how grommet tubes can have life-changing benefits, especially for seniors with glue ear. It highlights the importance of being ready for and handling post-procedure care.

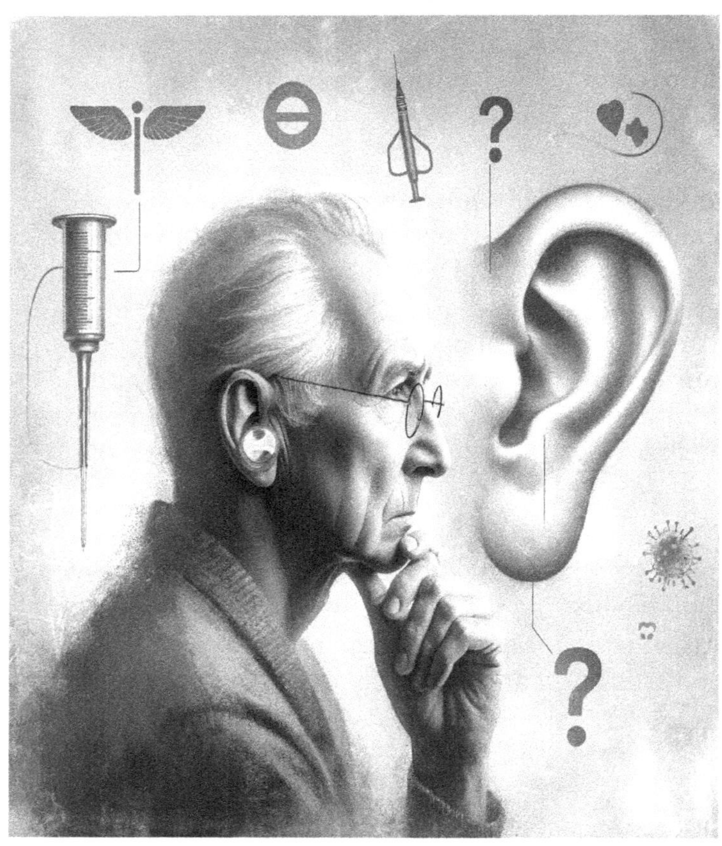

Seniors who are considering grommet tubes for glue ear need to understand the next steps. The initial step is to seek guidance from a healthcare professional, specifically an ENT specialist. These experts can thoroughly assess your ear health and determine if grommet tubes are right for you.

During the consultation, we will thoroughly discuss your medical history, current symptoms, and past treatments for glue ear. The ENT specialist might conduct various tests to evaluate your ear condition and the extent of fluid build-up, including hearing tests and tympanometry.

If grommet tubes are recommended, the ENT specialist will discuss the procedure, risks, and expected outcomes. They're available to address any questions or concerns you may have, aiding in your decision-making process. When making a decision about this procedure, remember to take into account your overall health, age-related factors, and lifestyle.

Audiologists are also essential during the post-procedure phase.st with hearing assessments and provide guidance on how to manage and maintain your hearing health once the tubes are in place.

Involving your primary care physician in the decision-making process is advantageous. Their input is valuable in understanding how the procedure aligns with your health plan and managing other conditions affecting your ear health.proceed with grommet tubes should be a collaborative one, made with the input of medical professionals who understand your unique health situation.

What About Metal Grommets?

Metal grommet tubes, also known as tympanostomy tubes, are indeed used in some cases for treating certain ear conditions, such as chronic otitis media (middle ear infections). These tubes are typically small and cylindrical and are inserted into a tiny incision in the eardrum to help ventilate the middle ear and prevent the accumulation of fluid. While most tympanostomy tubes are made from materials like silicone or plastic, metal tubes are also an option.

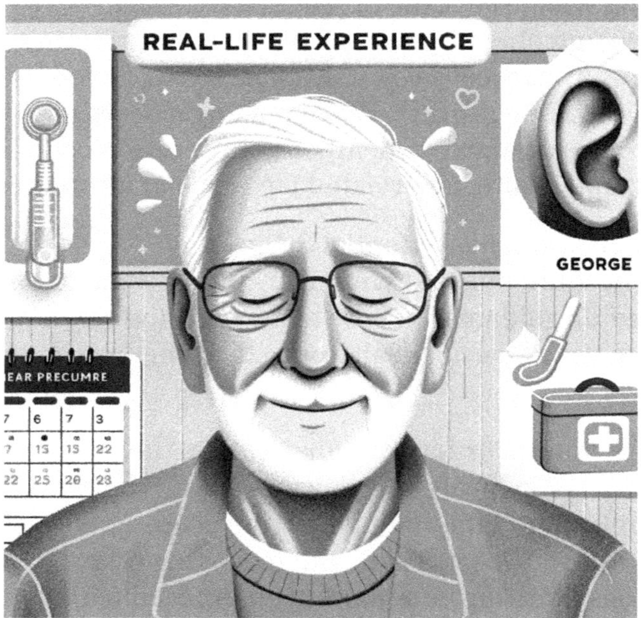

Safety and Efficacy:

- Biocompatibility: Metal tubes are usually made from materials like titanium, which are biocompatible and generally well-tolerated by the body.

- Durability: Metal tubes tend to be more durable than their plastic counterparts. They are less likely to become dislodged or require replacement, which can be a significant advantage in certain long-term treatments.
- Magnetic Resonance Imaging (MRI) Safety: One consideration with metal tubes is their interaction with MRI. While many modern metal tubes are designed to be MRI-safe, it's important to confirm this with the specific product used.

Considerations:

- Individual Suitability: The decision to use metal vs. plastic or silicone tubes depends on the individual case, the specific needs of the patient, and the physician's preference.
- Potential for Longer Retention: Metal tubes might be chosen in situations where longer-term ventilation of the middle ear is required. They are less likely to be extruded by the ear compared to non-metal tubes.
- Post-Surgical Care: As with any tympanostomy tube, appropriate post-insertion care is crucial to prevent infections or other complications.

Conclusion:

Metal grommet tubes can be a safe and effective option for the treatment of certain ear conditions, particularly in cases requiring longer-term ear ventilation. However, the choice of tube material should be made by an ENT specialist based on the specific medical needs and circumstances of the patient. If you or someone you know is considering tympanostomy tube insertion, it's important to discuss all available options, including the type of tube material, with a healthcare professional.

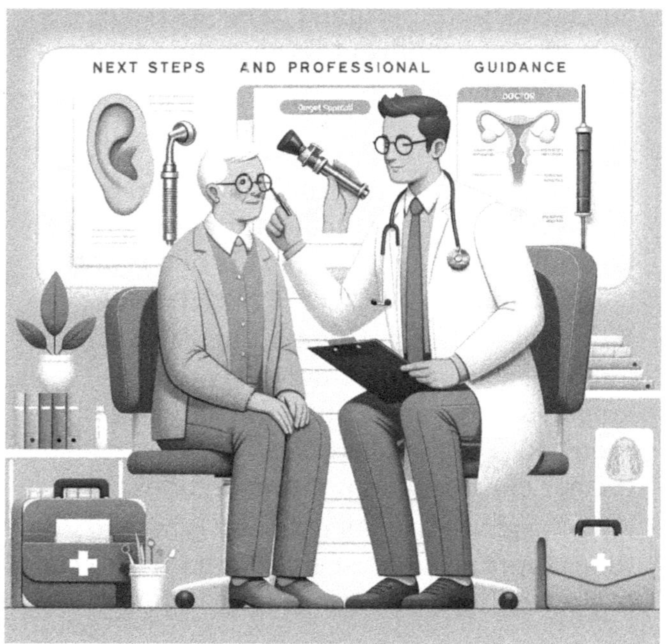

To sum up, grommet tubes have the potential to greatly benefit seniors with glue ear by improving their hearing and enhancing their quality of life. Personal experiences and professional advice shed light on the challenges and rewards of managing glue ear with grommet tubes.

A balanced approach involves considering the advantages and disadvantages while consulting healthcare experts. ENT specialists and audiologists are crucial in this process, providing their expertise and support. Patients should carefully evaluate the procedure, benefits, and risks before deciding on grommet tubes.e more than just a medical solution; they can be a gateway to staying connected with the world, engaging more fully in life's conversations, and enjoying the sounds that make life rich and fulfilling.

It's about reclaiming a part of oneself that glue ear's silence may have taken away.

Keep in mind that every person's situation is different, and the choice to pursue grommet tubes should be individualized, with guidance from trusted healthcare experts.

Bonus Chapter 3: Unclog your blocked ears with these 4 methods.

Imagine cotton balls stuffing your ears, not the soft kind but the annoying, sound-muffling type. That's ear congestion for you—uncomfortable, persistent, and downright frustrating. Dr. Melissa Gallagher, with her naturopathic wisdom, steps into the arena armed with nature's best to tackle this issue head-on. She outlines a simple, yet effective protocol designed to clear your ears and restore the harmony of sounds.

Step 1: Lubricate the Ear Joints

The Magic of Oil of Oregano

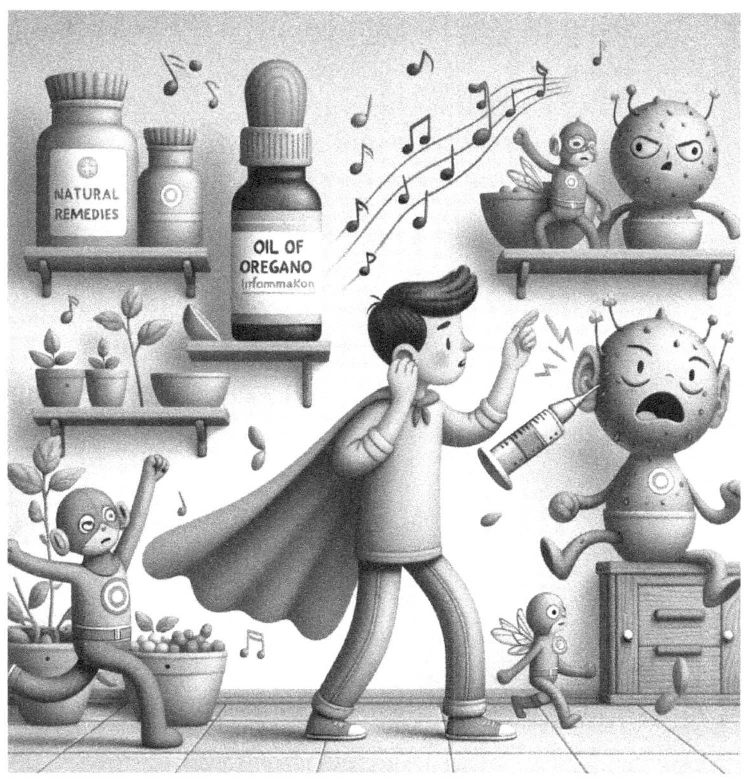

- **What's happening:** Your ear has three tiny bones, chilling like best buds in a hinge-like formation, crucial for transmitting sounds. But when fluid and inflammation crash the party, it's like throwing sand in the gears—everything gets stuck.

- **Dr. G's Solution:** Enter the oil of oregano, not just any oil, but a superhero in its own right. A few drops on the outer ear lobe and behind the ear start a chain reaction, breaking up fluid and telling inflammation it's time to pack up and leave.

- **Why It Works:** This oil's got the power to penetrate the skin and soothe the inflamed area, helping those tiny bones get back to their smooth moves.

Safety First! Remember, folks, the oil of oregano is potent. Mixing it with a carrier oil before application is like making sure your coffee has just the right amount of sugar—it's essential for the perfect experience.

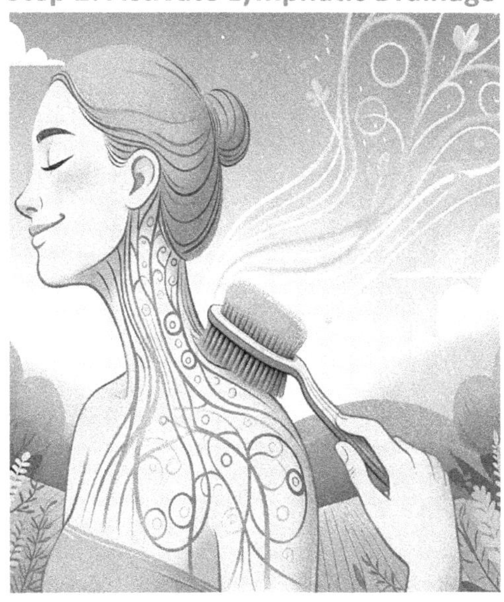

The Art of Dry Brushing and Lymphatic Massage

- **What's happening:** The lymphatic system is your body's unsung hero, working to remove toxins and excess fluids. When it's sluggish, everything backs up, including in your ears.

- **Dr. G's Strategy:** Grab a dry brush and brush the skin around your head, neck, and ears. Follow up with a soft lymphatic massage. It's like clearing traffic jams on the highway, making way for smooth sailing.

- **Why It Rocks:** This one-two punch stimulates lymphatic movement, reducing pressure and congestion. It's a natural detox for your ear area.

Clearing the Pathways with Neti Pots and Saline Sprays

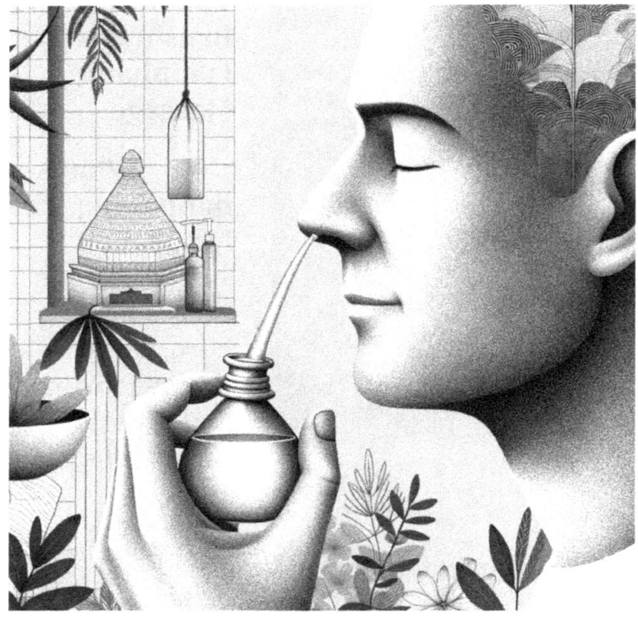

- **What's Happening:** Sinus congestion is like that one guest at the party who just won't leave, contributing to the whole ear congestion saga.

- **Dr. G's Game Plan:** Using a net pot or saline spray clears out the mucus and unwanted guests, reducing inflammation and irritation. It's like sending an eviction notice to congestion.

- **Pro Tip:** Enhancing net pot solutions with colloidal silver might just be the secret sauce for added anti-inflammatory and immune-boosting effects.

The Power of Ginger and Turmeric Tea

- **What's Happening:** Inflammation is the root of many evils, including ear congestion. It's the body's way of saying, "I'm working on it," but sometimes it overdoes it.
- **Dr. G's Secret Weapon:** Ginger and turmeric tea. These aren't just tasty beverages; they're inflammation's kryptonite. sipping on these teas can help soothe the ear, nose, and throat region, keeping the fluid at bay.
- **Why It's Awesome:** Beyond their comforting warmth, these teas pack a punch against inflammation, thanks to their natural compounds. It's like cozying up with a blanket that also fights ear congestion.

Boosting the Immune System and Minimizing Pathogenic Exposure

- **Beyond the Steps:** Dr. Gallagher doesn't stop at four steps; she offers a fifth—bolstering your immune system and reducing exposure to pathogens. It's about building a fortress around your health.

- **Why It Matters:** Strengthening your immune system is like having an elite team of bodyguards; it keeps potential threats at bay, preventing future ear congestion episodes.

Following Dr. Gallagher's guide is like tuning an instrument—each step brings you closer to the perfect harmony of health. It's not just about unclogging ears; it's about embracing a lifestyle that prioritizes natural remedies and the body's innate ability to heal. So, try it, stay consistent, and remember—nature has a fantastic way of hitting the right notes, especially for health.

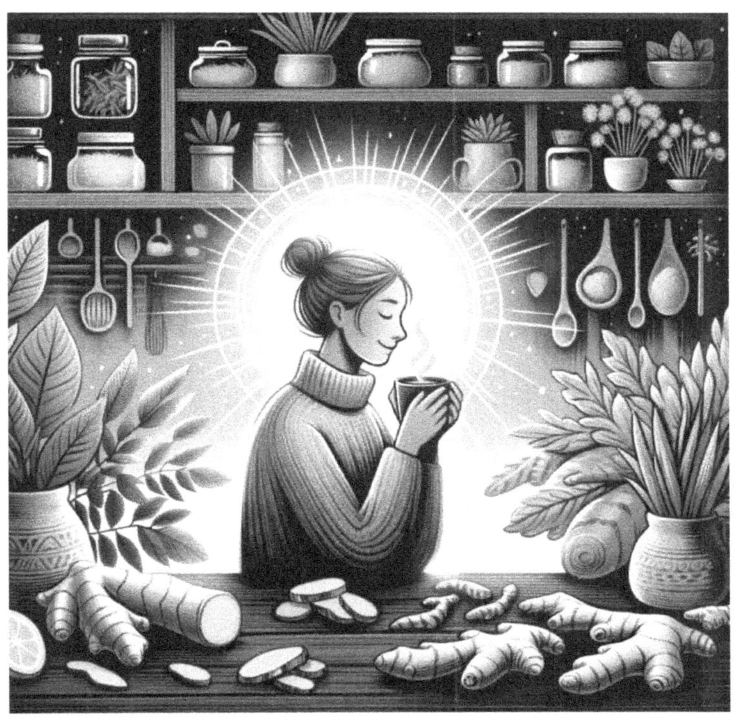

Dr. Gallagher's approach is more than just a temporary fix; it's a testament to the power of natural healing. By incorporating these steps into your daily routine, you're not just clearing your ears; you're opening yourself up to a world of holistic health benefits. Whether you're a skeptic or a believer in naturopathy, there's no denying the simplicity and effectiveness of this protocol. So, why not dive in? Your ears—and your overall well-being—might just thank you for it.

YouTube video resource:
https://www.youtube.com/watch?v=Jb61kq4bxbk

Bonus Chapter 3: What Else Could Help

Have you ever experienced that annoying feeling of ear fullness, where it seems like you're hearing the world through a thick blanket? Or maybe you've encountered a persistent clicking and ringing that's as unwelcome as a mosquito buzzing in your ear at night. These symptoms can be more than just bothersome; they can significantly affect your quality of life. But fear not! Today, we're going to unpack the mysteries of Eustachian Tube Dysfunction (ETD), a common culprit behind these symptoms, and explore practical exercises and acupressure techniques to find relief.

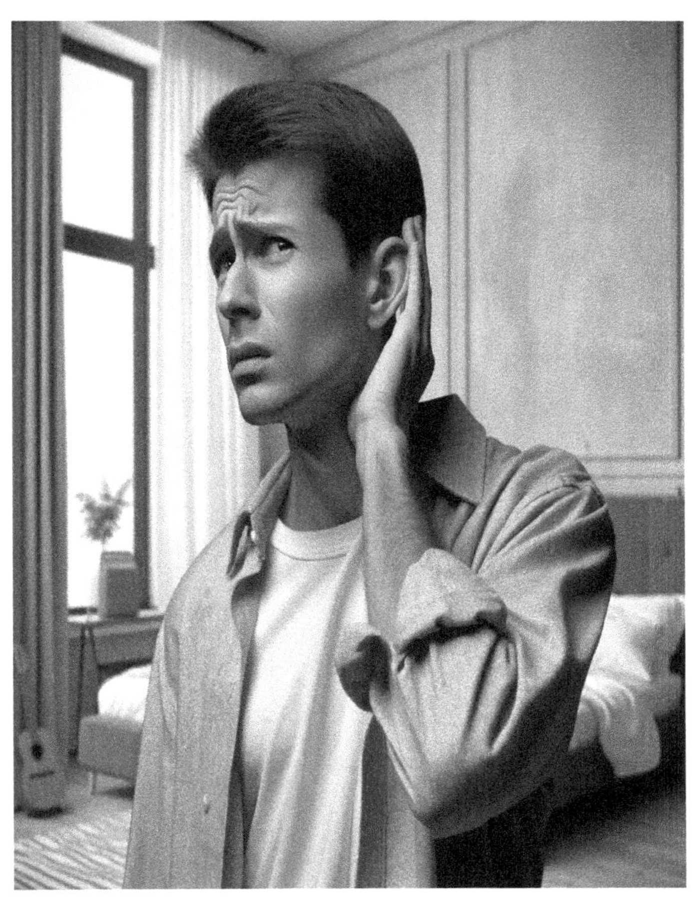

What's Up With My Ears? The Eustachian Tube Explained.

First off, let's talk about what the Eustachian tube does. Picture it as your ear's personal pressure regulator, balancing the air pressure on both sides of your eardrum. When it's not doing its job correctly because of inflammation, allergies, or other factors, you might experience ear fullness, clicking, and ringing. It's like your ears way of saying, "Hey, something's not right here!"

Rolling Up Our Sleeves: Exercises for ETD

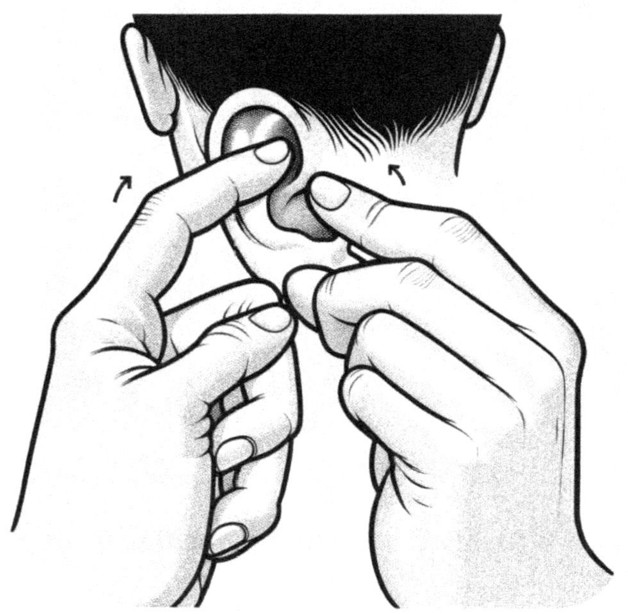

Behind-the-Ear Slide

- **What to do:** Simply place your fingers behind your ears and gently slide them down toward your neck. This can help get things moving and improve fluid dynamics.
- **Why it works:** It's all about encouraging drainage and movement in an area that's prone to getting sluggish.

Open-Mouth Jaw Moves

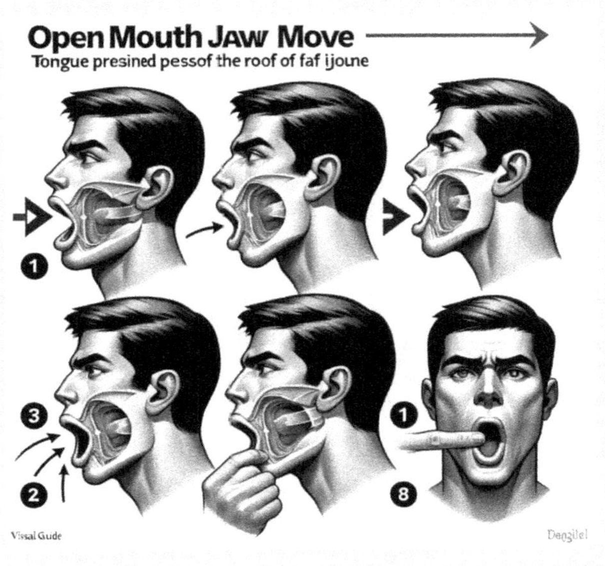

- **What to do:** Open your mouth about a finger's width and press your tongue to the roof of your mouth, then swallow. You might hear some crackling, which is a good sign!
- **Why it works:** This exercise targets the muscles and structures around the Eustachian tube, promoting opening and better drainage.

Tongue and Ear Coordination

- **What to do:** Combine tongue movements with gentle ear pulling to encourage the Eustachian tubes to open.

- **Why it works:** This quirky combo can help relieve pressure and promote fluid movement in the ear.

Pressing for Relief: Acupressure Techniques

Tragus Twist

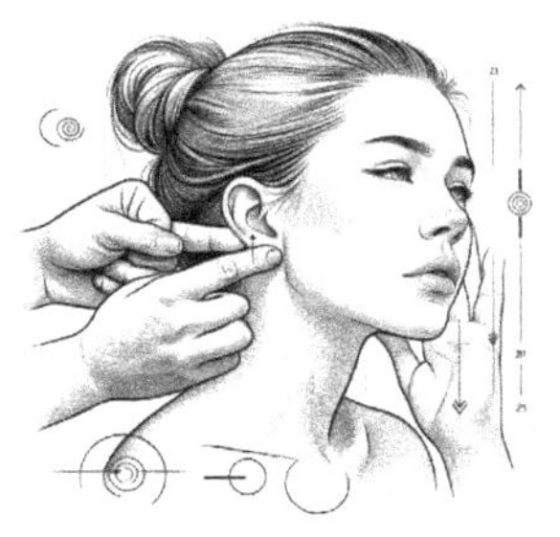

- **What to do:** Gently press and massage the tragus (the little of cartilage at the front of your ear canal) while opening and closing your mouth.
- **Why it works:** It's believed to help stimulate areas connected to the Eustachian tube, reducing discomfort.

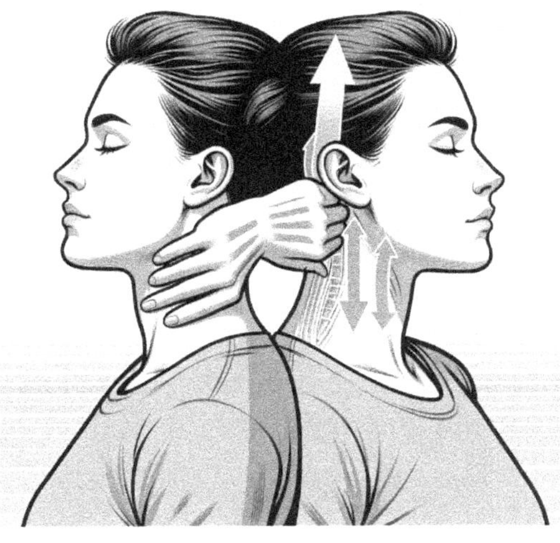

Neck Stretches

- **What to do:** Tilt your head to

one side, stretching the neck, then repeat on the other side.

- **Why it works:** These stretches can help reduce tension in the muscles around the Eustachian tubes, promoting better function.

Adding It All Up

Incorporating these exercises and acupressure techniques into your daily routine can offer significant relief for those suffering from ETD. Remember, consistency is key. Just like any other aspect of health, taking care of your ears is a daily commitment.

A Word of Caution

While these methods can provide relief, it's crucial to listen to your body. If you experience severe pain, bleeding, or other concerning symptoms, it's time to consult a healthcare professional. Your ears are precious; treat them with care.

Conclusion: Your Ears, Your Health

In the journey to better ear health, understanding the role of the Eustachian tube and how to support its function is crucial. With a blend of exercises and acupressure techniques, you can take proactive steps to ease discomfort and improve your quality of life. So, why wait? Start today, and let's turn down the volume on ear fullness, clicking, and ringing. Your ears—and your peace of mind—will thank you.

Learn more at:
https://www.youtube.com/watch?v=Pw4qzij-ryE

Bonus Chapter 4: Comprehensive Understanding of Tinnitus and Glue Ear.

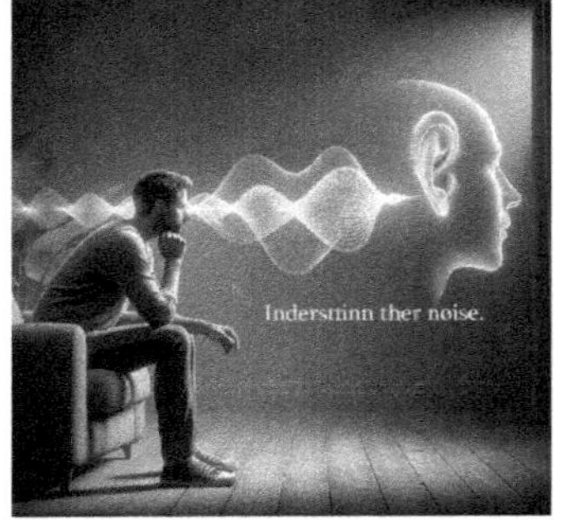

Imagine this: you're trying to enjoy a quiet moment, but there's a constant ringing in your ears that just won't quit. That's tinnitus for you—a condition that can range from a mild annoyance to a significant disruption in daily life. Now, add a glue ear into the mix, a condition where fluid builds up behind the eardrum, causing hearing loss and, sometimes, contributing to the development of tinnitus. These two are not just ear issues; they're significant barriers to clear hearing and peace of mind.

But why do they happen, and what's the link between them? Tinnitus often results from damage to the tiny hair cells in the inner ear, leading to those persistent sounds. Glue ear is usually because of Eustachian tube dysfunction, preventing proper drainage of fluid from the middle ear. When glue ear affects hearing, it can sometimes exacerbate or highlight the symptoms of tinnitus, making the sounds more noticeable.

In our journey today, we're diving deep into understanding these conditions and exploring practical, immediate relief methods. We're not just talking about coping strategies; we're focusing on actions you can take right now, in the comfort of your home, to bring some much-needed silence. Ready to turn down the volume on that internal noise? Let's get started.

Quick Relief Exercises for Tinnitus

When tinnitus flares up, the need for quick relief becomes paramount. Here's a practical approach designed to dial down the ringing in no time:

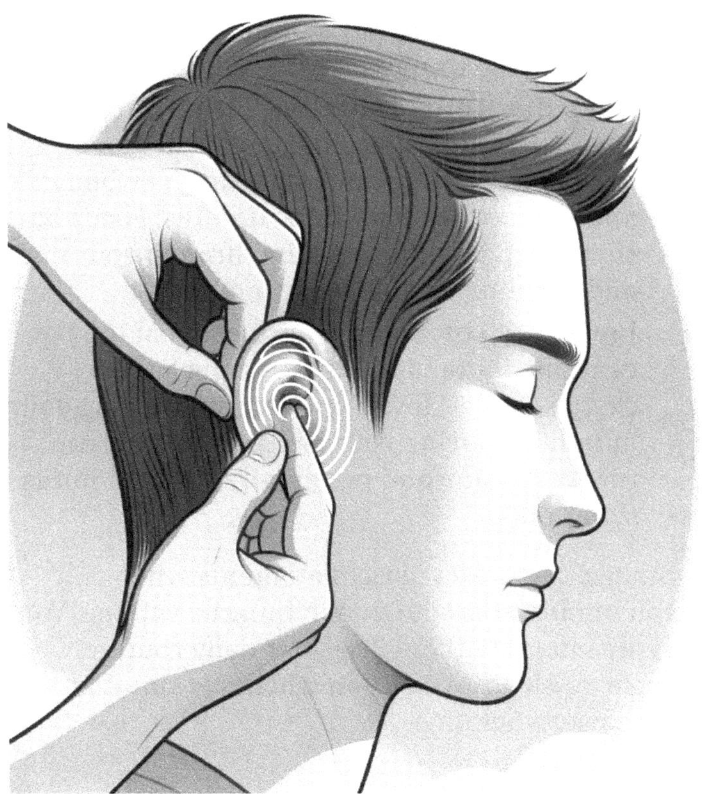

1. **Earlobe Massages**: Gently massaging your earlobes can increase blood circulation and may provide immediate relief. Use a soft, circular motion for about 30 seconds on each ear.
2. **Finger Drumming Technique**: This involves placing your hands over your ears with your fingers resting gently on the back of your head. Tap your index fingers against your skull to create a drumming sound. This method aims to reset your ear's perception, potentially quieting the tinnitus temporarily.
3. **Deep Breathing Exercises**: Stress often exacerbates tinnitus. Engaging in deep, mindful breathing can help relax your body and reduce the intensity of tinnitus. Focus on slow, deep breaths, inhaling through your nose and exhaling through your mouth.
4. **Jaw Exercises**: Sometimes tension in the jaw can contribute to tinnitus. Simple jaw exercises, like slowly opening and closing your mouth or moving your jaw side-to-side, can relieve tension and potentially lessen tinnitus symptoms.

You can use these exercises in moments when you need an immediate reduction in tinnitus volume. You can easily integrate them into your daily routine, offering a quick go-to solution whenever tinnitus becomes overwhelming.

For those seeking a more enduring solution to tinnitus, integrating certain exercises into your daily routine can be a game-changer. You can focus on these exercises to address some of the root causes of tinnitus, such as tension in the muscles around the jaw, neck, and shoulders, and improve overall ear health.

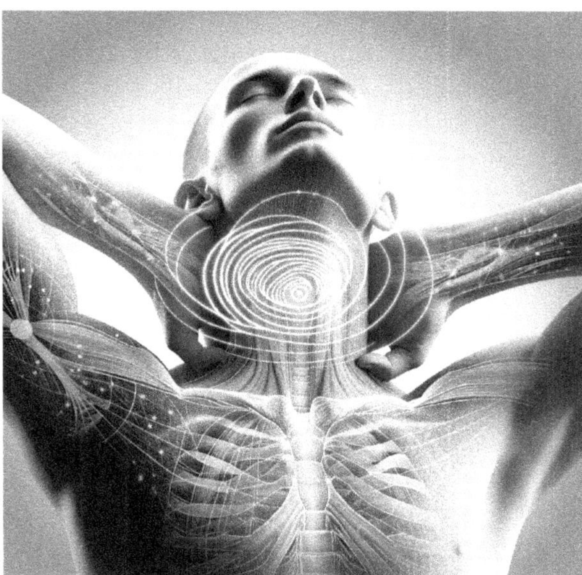

Here are some specific neck and shoulder stretches that can help relieve tension and potentially ease the exacerbation of tinnitus:

Keep your shoulders relaxed and avoid any tension in your neck and upper back. Breathe deeply and focus on the sensation of stretching and releasing any tightness or stiffness in your neck muscles. As you perform the neck rolls, be mindful of your range of motion and only go as far as feels comfortable for you. Remember to move slowly and smoothly, allowing the muscles to gradually loosen up. If you experience any pain or discomfort, reduce the range of motion or stop the exercise altogether. Neck rolls can help to improve flexibility, release tension, and promote relaxation in the neck and upper back area. They are especially beneficial for those who spend long hours sitting or working at a desk. Incorporate this exercise into your daily routine to maintain a healthy and mobile neck.1. Neck Rolls: Start by sitting or standing in a comfortable position with your spine straight. Slowly lower your chin towards your chest and rotate your head in a circular motion. As you roll your head to the right, gently stretch your neck by trying to touch your right ear to your right shoulder. Continue the circular motion, bringing your head back to the center and then rolling it to the left side. Repeat this exercise for several repetitions, moving slowly and with no pain or discomfort.

2. Shoulder Shrugs: Stand with your feet shoulder-width apart and relax your arms by your sides. Lift your shoulders up towards your ears, as if you're trying to touch them. Hold this position for a few seconds and then release, allowing your shoulders to drop back down. Repeat this movement for several repetitions, focusing on the upward and downward motion of your shoulders.

Incorporating these gentle neck rolls and shoulder shrugs into your daily routine can help improve blood circulation, reduce muscle tension, and provide relief from the exacerbation of tinnitus. However, it is important to consult with a healthcare professional or a physical therapist before starting any new exercise routine, especially if you have any pre-existing neck or shoulder conditions.

1. To perform a temporal muscle massage, start by locating the muscle on the side of the head. It is located just above the temple area and extends towards the back of the head. Using your fingertips or the pads of your thumbs, apply gentle pressure to the muscle. Start with small circular motions and accumulate the pressure as needed. Focus on any areas that feel tense or tender. Massage the muscle for about 5 to 10 minutes, or until you feel a sense of relaxation and relief. This massage technique helps to improve blood circulation in the area, release muscle tension, and ease any discomfort that may contribute to tinnitus. It is important to remember to be gentle and not to apply excessive pressure, as the area can be sensitive. If you experience any pain or discomfort during the massage, stop immediately and consult a healthcare professional.

2. Another exercise to open the Eustachian tubes is called the Toynbee maneuver. To perform this exercise, you need to pinch your nose shut

and swallow simultaneously. This action helps to regulate the pressure inside the middle ear and can relieve symptoms of Eustachian tube dysfunction, including tinnitus. The Valsalva maneuver can also be helpful. This exercise involves closing your mouth, pinching your nose shut, and gently blowing air through your nose, as if you were trying to inflate a balloon. These exercises help to promote the movement of air in and out of the Eustachian tubes, reducing any blockages and potentially easing tinnitus symptoms. It is important to consult with a healthcare professional before attempting any exercises to ensure they are safe and suitable for your specific condition.

3. Besides yoga, meditation, and guided imagery, there are several other relaxation techniques that can be effective in managing tinnitus-related stress. Deep breathing exercises, progressive muscle relaxation, and mindfulness techniques can all help to calm the mind and body, reducing stress levels and promoting a sense of relaxation. These techniques work by redirecting the focus away from the tinnitus sounds and towards a state of inner peace and tranquility. Regular practice of these relaxation techniques can also help improve sleep quality, as sleep disturbances are often associated with tinnitus. Incorporating these techniques into a daily routine can be beneficial in not only reducing

stress but also in improving overall well-being and coping with tinnitus symptoms.

Incorporating these exercises into your life can not only provide relief from tinnitus but also contribute to a healthier, more balanced lifestyle. Patience and consistency are key, as these methods aim to offer long-term relief rather than immediate fixes.

Conclusion: A Journey Towards Quieter Days

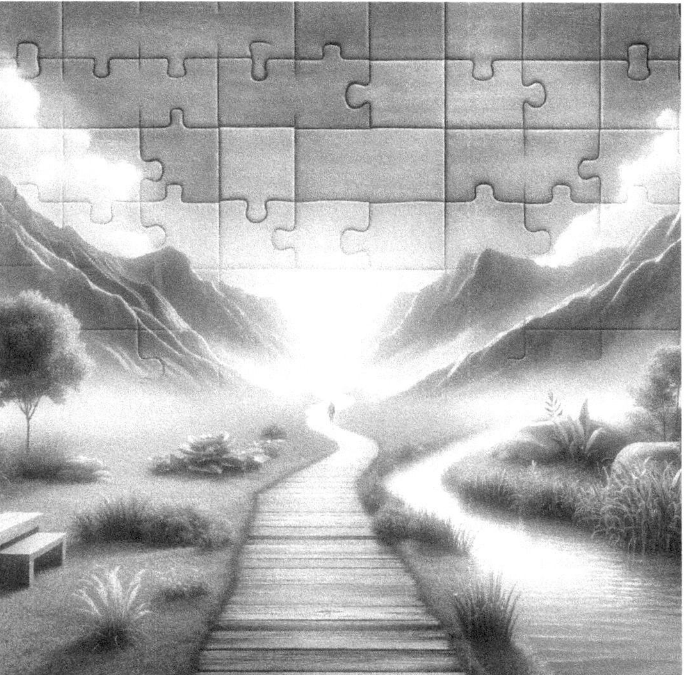

Embarking on the journey to manage tinnitus is a testament to your resilience. By incorporating quick relief and long-lasting exercises into your daily life, you're taking proactive steps toward quieter, more peaceful days. Remember, the key to these exercises is consistency and patience; improvements may come gradually. As you continue to practice these techniques, you're not just seeking relief; you're also enhancing your overall well-being and quality of life. Keep one day at a time, and know that every slight effort is a step towards a significant change.

Resources

Struggling with glue ear? Discover a natural path to relief with SharpEar, a unique supplement blending traditional wisdom with modern science.

Why SharpEar?

- Targeted Support: Specifically formulated to address glue ear by nurturing your ear's health.
- Natural Ingredients: SharpEar is packed with vitamins and herbal extracts known for their auditory benefits.
- Safety and Purity: Produced in FDA-registered facilities, ensuring the highest quality and safety standards.

Learn More

Curious about how SharpEar can specifically help with glue ear? Click here for detailed information and discover a natural solution to your auditory challenges.

Visit Here

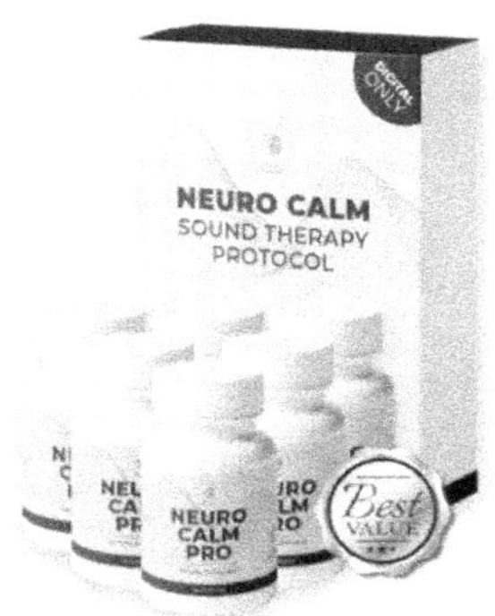

Neuro Calm Pro offers a natural approach to

managing glue ear with its blend of anti-inflammatory and nerve-supporting ingredients. It's designed to improve ear health, enhance ear-brain connections, and reduce symptoms like ear ringing. If you're seeking a holistic solution for glue ear, [click here](#) to learn how Neuro Calm Pro might help you regain clearer hearing and overall ear health.

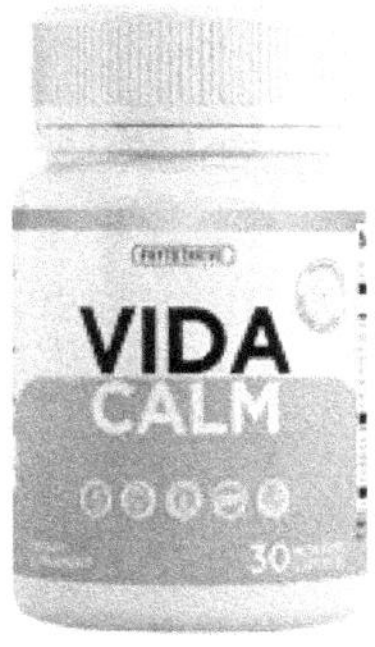

Struggling with tinnitus or glue ear? Discover

Relief with VidaCalm, a supplement combining herbs and nutrients to support healthy hearing. VidaCalm targets the root causes of tinnitus, ensuring a healthier auditory system. Made in an FDA-approved facility, it's 100% natural and side effect free. Experience the benefits of improved hearing and overall ear health. To learn more about how VidaCalm can aid in your hearing wellness journey, click here.

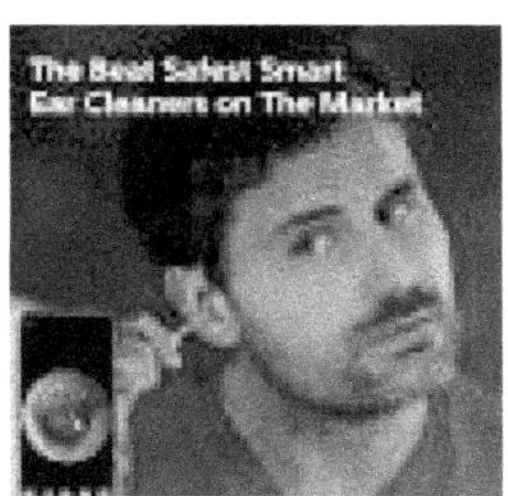

Discover Ear Health Like Never Before with EarOkay

If you're reading "Understanding Glue Ear: A Guide For All Ages," you know how crucial ear health is. But did you know that maintaining ear cleanliness is a key part of managing glue ear? That's where EarOkay comes in!

EarOkay: A Revolution in Ear Care

- Gentle and Effective: Specially designed to be safe and efficient for ear cleaning.
- Enhanced Ear Health: Regular use can help prevent the buildup of wax and debris, common culprits in glue ear.

Why Choose EarOkay?

- Innovative Design: Tailored for comfortable and thorough ear cleaning.
- Trusted by Experts: Recommended by healthcare professionals.

Embark on your journey to better ear health with EarOkay. It's more than just cleaning; it's about giving your ears the care they deserve. Click here to explore how EarOkay can be a vital part of your ear health regimen

Does your salad contain this vegetable?

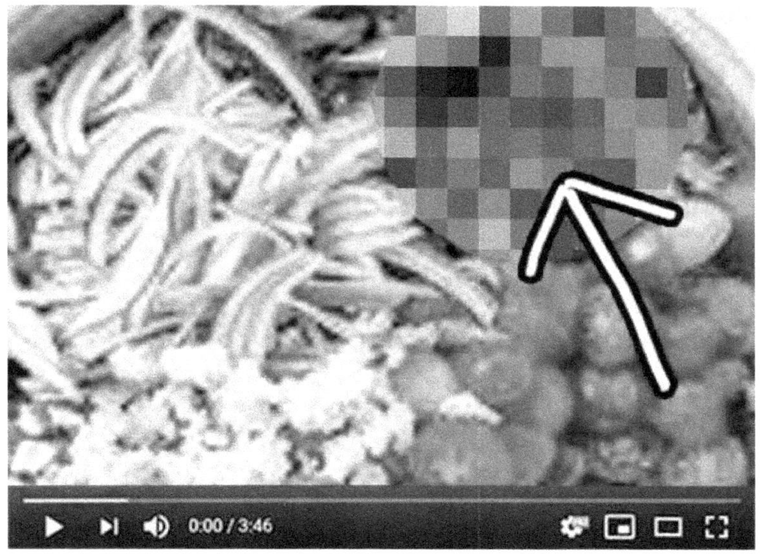

New research out of the University of Verona, Italy found an ingredient called lectin found inside this so-called "healthy" vegetable will **poke holes in your gut**, the lining of your intestine...

meaning it cannot absorb nutrients, increasing inflammation and slowing your metabolism, making you fatter and sicker.

Researchers found lectin is so dangerous its now referred to as a "anti-nutrient"...

And it's found in **this everyday vegetable**.

Yes it sounds crazy.

I thought that too, but then I saw this alarming video.

So what is this evil vegetable?

>>> Click Here To Discover The One Vegetable You Should NEVER Eat (Makes You Fat And Sick

About This Author

Author Bio: Jagoda E. Handor

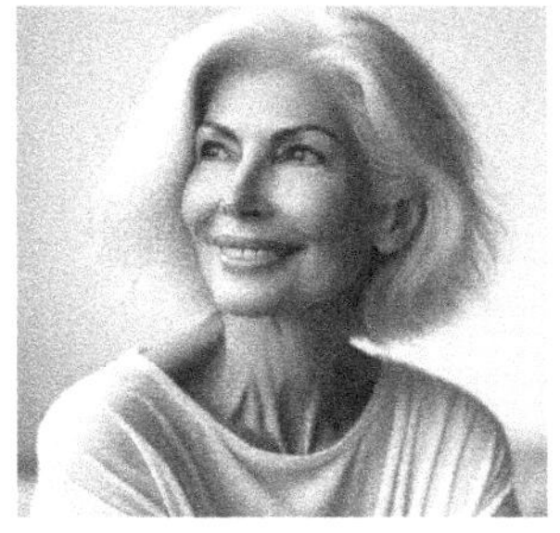

In the vibrant tapestry of life, Jagoda E. Handor's story stands out as a testament to resilience, learning, and empowerment. A British woman in her 60s, Jagoda's journey through health an

wellness is as inspiring as it is instructive. Having grappled with a myriad of health challenges throughout her life, including persistent ear infections, candida, and osteoporosis, Jagoda has become a beacon of hope and wisdom for those seeking a path to better health

Jagoda's early years were marked by frequent visits to doctors and specialists, as she navigated the complexities of her health conditions. Candida, a particularly stubborn adversary, brought with it a host of issues that impacted her quality of life. However, Jagoda's spirit, undeterred by these challenges, propelled her on a quest for knowledge and healing

Through her relentless pursuit, she learned from some of the best health experts, absorbing their teachings and applying them to her life. Her journey wasn't just about finding treatments; it was about transforming her lifestyle. Jagoda embraced a holistic approach to health, discovering that the key to wellness lies as much in prevention and lifestyle choices as it does in medical care

Now in her 60s, Jagoda is a living example of how adopting simple yet effective health strategies can bring about profound changes. Her experience with managing osteoporosis, ear infections, and candida has equipped her with invaluable insights into the importance of diet, exercise, stress management, and natural remedies

In her writings, Jagoda invites readers of all ages to join her in this journey of health and self-discovery. She shares not just her knowledge, but her personal stories of struggles and triumphs, making her advice relatable and encouraging. Her message is clear and compelling: it's never too late to clean up your health, and the simplest changes can often make the most significant impact

Jagoda E. Handor isn't just an author; she's a mentor and friend, guiding you through the ups and downs of health management with empathy, experience, and enthusiasm. Join her, and discover how you too can embark on a path to a healthier, happier life, no matter your age or challenges

Free Gift

5 Step. 5 Minute Balance Exercises For Seniors Over 80 - The 1st 7 Days

As well as to be notified on any new releases, giveaways, contests, cover reveals and so much more.

Click here to sign up for my newsletter

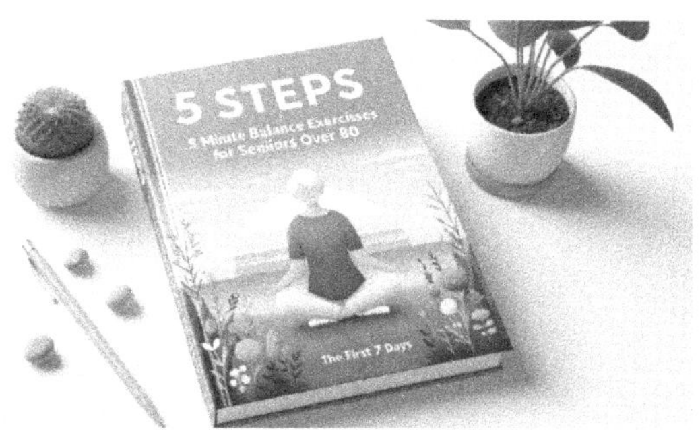

Click here to sign up for my newsletter

Review This Book

P.S. It Means the world to me that you brought my book. Writing is my passion and I look forward to YOUR feedback.

So if you liked this book, I'd like to ask for a small favor. Would you be so kind to leave a review on Amazon? It'd be very much appreciated!

From your friend, Jagoda Elka. Handor

www.ingramcontent.com/pod-product-compliance
Lightning Source LLC
Chambersburg PA
CBHW070812280726
48660CB00015B/409